MEDICAL
INTELLIGENCE
UNIT

ARTIFICIAL CHORDAE IN MITRAL VALVE SURGERY

Claudio Zussa, M.D., F.C.C.P.

Treviso Regional Hospital
Treviso, Italy

R.G. LANDES COMPANY
AUSTIN

MEDICAL INTELLIGENCE UNIT

ARTIFICIAL CHORDAE IN MITRAL VALVE SURGERY

R.G. LANDES COMPANY
Austin

CRC Press is the exclusive worldwide distributor of publications of the Medical Intelligence Unit.
CRC Press, 2000 Corporate Blvd., NW, Boca Raton, FL 33431. Phone: 407/994-0555.

Submitted: December 1993
Published: April 1994

Production Manager: Terry Nelson
Copy Editor: Constance Kerkaporta

Please address all inquiries to the Publisher:
R.G. Landes Company, 909 Pine Street, Georgetown, TX 78626
or
P.O. Box 4858, Austin, TX 78765
Phone: 512/ 863 7762; FAX: 512/ 863 0081

ISBN 1-879702-97-5
CATALOG # LN0297

Library of Congress Cataloging-in-Publication Data
Zussa, Claudio.
Artificial chordae in mitral valve surgery / Claudio Zussa.
p. cm. -- (Medical intelligence unit)
ISBN 1-8789702-97-5 (hardcover) :
1. Mitral valve--Surgery. 2. Heart valve prosthesis. 3. Chordae tendineae--Surgery.
I. Title. II. Series.
[DNLM: 1. Mitral valve--surgery. 2. Heart Valve Prosthesis.
3. Chordae Tendineae--surgery. WG 262 296a 1994]
RD598.35.H42Z87 1994
617.4' 12059--dc20
DNLM/DLC
for Library of Congress 94-9194 CIP

While the authors, editors and publisher believe that drug selection and dosage and the specifications and usage of equipment and devices, as set forth in this book, are in accord with current recommendations and practice at the time of publication, they make no warranty, expressed or implied, with respect to material described in this book. In view of the ongoing research, equipment development, changes in governmental regulations and the rapid accumulation of information relating to the biomedical sciences, the reader is urged to carefully review and evaluate the information provided herein.

CONTENTS

INTRODUCTION

The goal of cardiac valve surgery is to restore satisfactory heart function so the patient can assume an active life, regardless of age.[1]

Many factors are critical in achieving this result. First of all the timing of operation, a well-chosen and and well-executed surgical procedure, including use of the "best" available valve device, if needed; correct counseling and follow-up of the patient by both surgeon and referring cardiologist and an effective rehabilitation program.

Timing and choice of operation are closely related. A cardiologist would be reluctant to refer a patient, still functionally intact, for surgery without an "optimal" surgical solution for his valve disease.[2] Yet, in our opinion, inserting a prosthetic valve to improve cardiac function, changes the pathological state but doesn't cure it. At the very least, the prospect of reoperation—in the case of a biological valve prosthesis—or the discomfort and the complications related to anticoagulant therapy—in case of a mechanical prosthesis—diminish the quality of the patient's life.

Patients who have undergone valve replacement suffer from psychological problems arising from the procedure, from the fear of carrying a "foreign body" in their heart to anxiety associated with the sounds of mechanical valve prostheses.[3] Moreover, the classic procedure for valve prosthesis insertion reduces left ventricular performance due to interruption of annulus-ventricle continuity.

Many options are available to treat aortic valve disease, e.g, pulmonary autografts, homografts, free-hand reconstruction of the cusps with different materials, and stentless pericardial or porcine bioprostheses, in addition to conservative procedures and the traditional biological and mechanical prostheses. Yet for disease in the mitral position there are few alternatives to conservative treatment or to valve replacement with classic biological or mechanical prostheses (free-hand stentless pericardial valves, mitral homografts). For these reasons many techniques have been proposed to improve the results of mitral valve repair.

Problems of the mitral annulus have been moreorless satisfactorily addressed. Treatment of dilatation and deformity of the annulus is well-established, e.g, simple sutures or plications, pericardium-reinforced sutures, different prosthetic rings. The treatment of leaflet pathology—fibrosis, calcification, shrinkage, perforation—is still unsolved. It requires development of biocompatible tissues for leaflet extension or partial replacement. Yet I believe the weak point in mitral repair is still the subvalvular apparatus.

Indeed at least 30% of patients referred for mitral pathology could not have their valves satisfactory repaired with the usual techniques due to involvement of the subvalvular apparatus.

Cardiac surgeons realize that a mitral valve with degenerative pathology cannot be successfully repaired with traditional techniques because the subvalvular apparatus is extensively damaged, as in cases of degeneration with thinning and elongation of most of the chordae tendineae, or elongation of fine chordae arising from thin and sessile papillary muscles (fibroelastic deficiency), or multiple anterior and posterior chordal rupture, or almost complete flail of one leaflet. This frustrating experience has stimulated research to find new ways for the surgeon to apply his skill to treat this set of patients. And this is, in fact, a large group of patients. Mitral prolapse is the most common valve disorder in the Western world; the prevalence is 19-24%.[4]

The need for chordal substitutes for some patients undergoing open-heart mitral valve surgery has long been recognized.[5] The development of reliable—but imperfect—prosthetic valves reduced the interest of many cardiac surgeons in valve repair. Yet experimental and clinical studies have demonstrated that appropriate mitral valve repair is better than any available prosthesis. These findings revived interest in developing techniques and materials to improve the results of mitral valve surgery.

This book describes the result of our experimental and clinical experience with artificial mitral valve chordae substitutes. It is dedicated to Dr. Robert W.M. Frater who, as a young Fellow at the beginning of open-heart mitral valve repair, was deeply involved in the development of new techniques and is a friendly teacher and a stimulating researcher today.

References

1. Walter PJ, Mohan R, Amsel BJ: Quality of life after heart valve replacement. J Heart Valve Dis 1992; 1:34-41.
2. Barlow JB: Idiopathic (degenerative) and rheumatic mitral valve prolapse: historical aspects and an overview. J Heart Valve Dis 1992; 1:163-74.
3. Limb D, Kay PH, Murday AJ: Problems associated with mechanical heart valve sounds. Eur J Cardiothorac Surg 1992; 6:618-20.
4. Cheng TO: Mitral valve prolapse. Disease-a-month 1987; 33:486-534.
5. Frater RWM, Berghuis J, Brown AL et al: The experimental and clinical use of autogenous pericardium for the replacement and extension of mitral and tricuspid valve cusps and chordae. J Cardiovasc Surg (Torino) 1965; 6:214-28.

ACKNOWLEDGMENT

I would like to thank everyone who shared with me this exciting experience.

The experimental phase of this work could not have been done without the technical skills of A. Leon, P. Bon, F. Rivera and F. Wasserman from the laboratory of the Department of Cardiothoracic Surgery of the Albert Einstein College of Medicine of New York.

The clinical experience was greatly endorsed by the Chief of the Department of Cardiac Surgery of Treviso Regional Hospital, Dr. Carlo Valfré.

Dr. Marco Galloni, from the Veterinary Medical School of Turin University, deserves particular thanks for the support of his longstanding friendship and the superb work examining anatomical specimens and preparing most of the illustrations in this book.

Finally I would like to thank all of my coworkers at the Cardiac Surgery Department of Treviso Regional Hospital who share with me the enthusiasm for this new technique.

CHAPTER 1

HISTORICAL PERSPECTIVE

The description of the stethoscope by Laennec in 1819 represented a major step in the scientific approach to the heart. Auscultation joined observation, inspection, palpation and percussion in the process of understanding cardiac pathophysiology during life.[1] Cardiac sounds and murmurs could be correlated to the clinical status of the patient and to the postmortem observations of valvular pathologies. The apical murmur produced by mitral regurgitation was identified (Hope, 1831), and in one patient it was correlated with chordal rupture (Williams, 1840) demonstrated at autopsy.[2]

Although the pathology of rheumatic mitral valve disease was described in the 19th century, it was only in 1944 that Bailey and Hickam[3] described the basic characteristics of the floppy mitral valve: redundant cusps, elongated and ruptured chordae, and dilated annulus. They excluded a rheumatic etiology by histological examination of postmortem specimens. But the histological aspects of the floppy mitral valve were only fully described by Fernex in 1958.[4] He established that mucoid degeneration of the connective tissue was the fundamental change in the floppy mitral valve, in cases without clinical evidence of systemic connective tissue pathology. This work was supported by Pomerance[5] and King,[6] who carefully compared normal and floppy mitral valves.

An similar comparison by Baker of normal, floppy non-regurgitant, and floppy regurgitant valves focused on the chordae tendineae. This study demonstrated mucoid connective tissue degeneration in floppy valve chordae as well.[7] The author suggested this degeneration was the etiology of chordal rupture, validating the observations of Hickey[8] and Jerasaty[9] regarding the frequent detection of ruptured chordae in floppy mitral valves. Moreover the gross appearance (elongation and thinning) and distribution to the leaflets of chordae were accurately described in surgical specimens of floppy and non-floppy mitral valves.[6,7]

Recently the subvalvular apparatus has been postulated to be one of the causes of "innocent" cardiac murmurs.[10] On echocardiography of 100 young men with this type of auscultatory finding, Onishchenko and Krylov demonstrated fluttering chordae in 37% of them. These structures had increased mobility due to their excessive length and weak tension, although no mitral regurgitation could be detected. A correlation with local papillary muscle dysfunction was also suggested.

One of the most significant contributions to the definition of the anatomical and clinical aspects of degenerative mitral valve disease was made by Barlow.[11] In a recent review of the literature of the last 30 years regarding this pathology the author[12] asserts that terms such as "billowing" and "prolapse" should be defined based on functional anatomy. "Billowing" is the exaggerated bulging of mitral leaflets into the left atrium during systole and "floppy" is the more advanced form of this phenomenon. Leaflets and chordae are affected, but the valve is still competent throughout systole. When in floppy valve leaflets no longer coapt, valve incompetence ensues. This condition is "prolapse". Advanced cases with chordal rupture and eversion of segments of the leaflets into the left atrium, is referred to as "flail."

Many hypotheses have been proposed to explain the relation between the floppy valve (leaflets and chordae degeneration) and altered left ventricular segmental contractility. Indeed a localized cardiomyopathy, producing loose chordae that lead to or increase leaflet redundancy, has been suggested,[13] A change in the subvalvular apparatus causing abnormal stretching of the ventricular wall has been proposed as well.[14]

Many aspects of the pathophysiology of mitral valve prolapse are still controversial. Moreover anatomic and functional changes produced by surgical treatment of this disease (valve repair or replacement) are not fully understood. Further research is necessary.

REFERENCES

1. Wooley CF, Baker PB, Kolibash AJ et al. The floppy, mixomatous mitral valve, mitral valve prolapse, and mitral regurgitation. Prog Cardiovasc Dis 1991; 33:397-433.

2. Keele KD. The application of physics of sound to 19th century cardiology: With particular reference to the part played by CJB Williams and James Hope. Clio Med. 1973; 8:191-221.

3. Bailey OT, Hickam JB. Rupture of mitral chordae tendineae. Am Heart J 1944; 28:578-600.

4. Fernex PM, Fernex C. La degenerescence mucoide des valvules mitrales. Ses repercussions fonctionnelles. Helv Medica Acta 1958; 25:694-705.

5. Pomerance A. Ballooning deformity (mucoid degeneration) of atrioventricular valves. Br Heart J 1969; 31:343-51.

6. King BD, Clark MA, Baba N et al. "Myxomatous" mitral valve: Collagen dissolution as the primary defect. Circulation 1982; 66:288-96.

7. Baker PB, Bansal GJ, Boudoulas H et al. Floppy mitral valve chordae tendineae: Histopathologic alterations. Hum Pathol 1988; 19:507-12.

8. Hickey AJ, Wilcken DEL, Wright JS et al. Primary (spontaneous) chordal rupture. Relation of mixomatous valve disease and mitral valve prolapse. J Am Coll Cardiol 1985; 5:1341-6.

9. Jerasaty RM, Edwards JE, Chawla SK. Mitral valve prolapse and ruptured chordae tendineae. Am J Cardiol 1985; 55:138-42.

10. Onishchenko EF, Krylov AA. The significance of the chordal apparatus of the heart in forming "innocent" murmurs (clinical echocardiographic research). Ter Arkh 1991; 63:17-22.

11. Barlow JB, Pocock WA, Marchand P et al. The significance of late systolic murmurs. Am Heart J 1963; 66:443-52.

12. Barlow JB. Idiopathic (degenerative) and rheumatic mitral valve prolapse: Historical aspects and an overview. J Heart Valve Dis 1992; 1:163-74.

13. Gulotta SJ, Gulco L, Padmanabhan V et al. The syndrome of systolic click, murmur and mitral valve prolapse—A cardiomyopathy? Circulation 1974; 49:717-28.

14. Devereux RB, Perloff JK, Reichek N et al. Mitral valve prolapse. Circulation 1976; 54:3-14.

CHAPTER 2

Surgical Anatomy

ANATOMY OF THE CHORDAE TENDINEAE

Considerable individual variations have been reported in number, branching and distribution of mitral valve chordae.[1-4] They originate from the papillary muscles (Fig. 2.1) and, after branching, they distribute to the ventricular aspect of the free edge (first order or marginal chordae) or to the ventricular surface (second order) of the leaflets attaching every few millimeters and leaving an unsupported area of 0.5-1 cm in the central part of the free edges (Fig. 2.2) of the anterior and posterior cusps (bare area). Chordae that, originating directly from the ventricular wall, support part of the posterior leaflet are defined as third order or mural chordae.[5] Other authors[6] refer to those arising from the papillary muscles and inserting into the valve annulus or the ventricular wall as tertiary chordae; the latter structures are called also false chordae or false tendons.

Analysis of the stress/strain characteristics of marginal versus basal chordae tendineae has demonstrated that the stress carried by the basal chordae is lower than that carried by the marginal ones, as a consequence of which the marginal cordae are stiffer than the basal chordae.[7] The ratio of papillary origins to leaflet insertions is, on average, 1 to 2,[5] and there are twice as many marginal as basal chordae.[7] The commissural valve tissue is supported by chordae originating at the apex of the papillary muscles (Fig. 2.3) and branching to both sides with the apical single branch reaching the commissure.[5-6]

Since the posterior leaflet is not a single structure, but is composed of at least three segments, Frater and co-workers[8] suggested a classification of mitral chordae based on the leaflet portion supported. This classification is very useful during valve repair to uneqivocally identify groups of chordae.

Looking from the atrium (Fig. 2.4) and starting clockwise from the anterolateral commissure, the authors defined chordae for:

(1) the anterolateral half of the anterior leaflet (from the commissure to the bare area of the anterior leaflet);

(2) the posteromedial half of the anterior leaflet;

(3) the posteromedial commissural cusp;

(4) the posteromedial half of the central component of the posterior leaflet (posteromedial component of the posterior cusp);

(5) the anterolateral half of the central component of the posterior leaflet (anterolateral component of the posterior leaflet;

(6) the anterolateral commissural cusp.

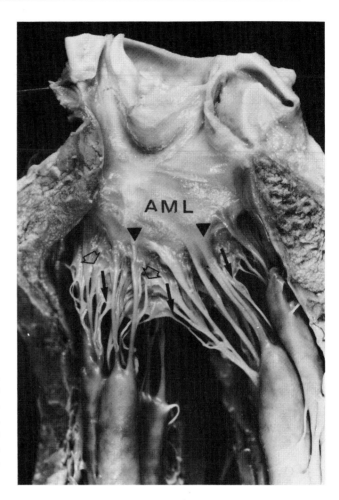

Fig. 2.1. Distribution of chordae tendineae. Originating from papillary muscles they branch to the free edge—first order—(black arrows), to the ventricular surface—second order—(empty arrows) of the leaflets and to the valve annulus (black triangles). AML=ventricular surface of the anterior mitral leaflet.

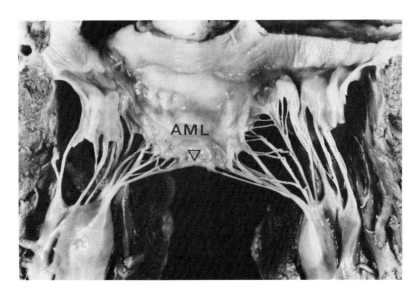

Fig. 2.2. After branching, first order chordae leave an unsupported area in the central part of each leaflet (empty triangle). AML=atrial surface of the anterior mitral leaflet.

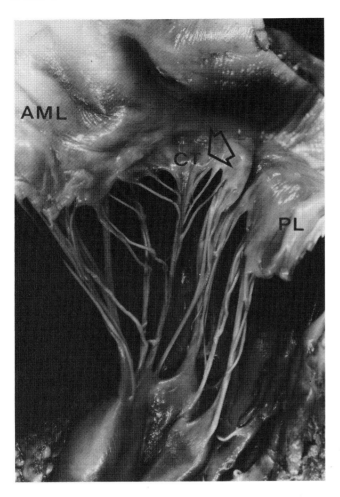

Fig. 2.3. Chordae arising from the tip of the papillary muscles branch to the commissural tissue (empty arrow). AML=anterior mitral leaflet; CT=commissural tissue; PL=posterior leaflet.

Fig. 2.4. Atrial view of the six normal components of the mitral leaflets. Large black arrow: anterolateral component of the anterior leaflet; large empty arrow: posteromedial component of the anterior leaflet; black triangle: posteromedial commissural tissue; small empty arrow: posteromedial component of the posterior leaflet; small black arrow: anterolateral component of the posterior leaflet; empty triangle: anterolateral commissural tissue; black square: central component of the posterior leaflet, often present in degenerated valves. AL=anterior leaflet; PL=posterior leaflet

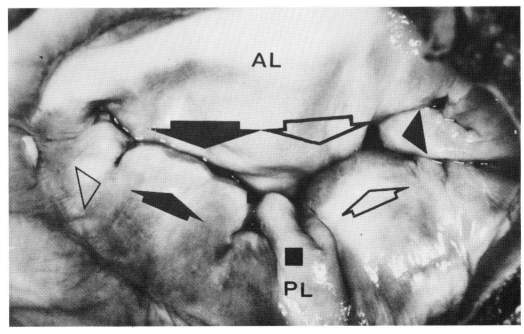

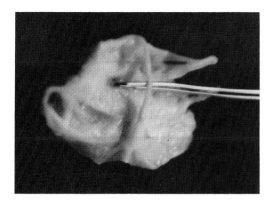

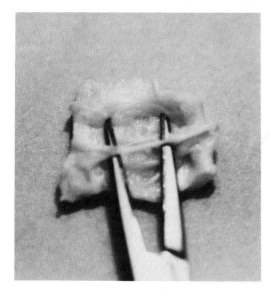

Fig. 2.5 A and B. Two typical cases in which abnormal chordae tendineae joint two points of the leaflet, without any connection with the papillary muscles, reducing leaflet support.

DEGENERATIVE CHORDAL PATHOLOGY

From the point of view of surgery, Frater and co-workers[8] identified three different types of chordal pathologies each possibly requiring different operative approaches:

(1) chordal rupture with normal cusps (trauma, myocardial infarction, endocarditis);

(2) chordal elongation and/or rupture with associated leaflet degeneration, as in the case of the floppy valve;

(3) chordal elongation associated with rheumatic cusp alterations.

With regard to the "normal" anatomy, the considerable variation in chordal distribution suggested that areas of the leaflets

not adequately supported by chordae might be a factor in the development of a floppy valve (Fig. 2.5). The hypothesis claims that weak support could lead to progressive deformity of these areas stressed by systolic closure pressure.[9]

Thinning and elongation—associated with areas of bulging—corresponding to large acid mucopolysaccharide deposits, are the most common pathological findings affecting floppy valve chordae (Fig. 2.6 and 2.7). Often cystic formations are present on the surface of leaflets (Fig. 2.8) and chordae (Fig. 2.9 and 2.10). Histologic examination confirms the mucopolysaccharide content of these structures (Fig. 2.11).

In a masterful study of the pathology of mitral incompetence, Edwards[10] described several features characteristic of the myxomatous mitral valve. Interchordal leaflet hooding or prolapse is the first (Fig. 2.6), resulting from the accumulation of myxomatous tissue in the spongiosa layer (the central part of the leaflet) that reaches the supportive fibrosa layer and produces weakening of the leaflet structure (Fig. 2.12). A second feature is that fibrotic changes, observed in some cases of myxomatous mitral valve, don't replace the normal components of the leaflet but rather are a fibrotic thickening of the contact surface layer (atrialis). Also commissures are not fused, contrary to what is normally observed in fibrous changes due to rheumatic pathology.

Chordal rupture (Fig. 2.13 and 2.14) is reported with a wide range of incidence in different series of surgical specimens. This is probably related to the variability of pathological changes and to the nonuniform timing of surgery.[11-21] In fact, analyzing the natural history of mitral regurgitation due to valve prolapse, Kolibash[18,22-23] reported a long period (average of 25 years) in which patients remained asymptomatic, although with a cardiac murmur. The progression from mild to severe mitral regurgitation associated with the onset of significant cardiac symptoms was related to chordal rupture in more than half of the cases.

Carpentier and co-workers made observations of particular interest to surgeons.[24] In cases of nonrheumatic mitral regurgitation they dis-

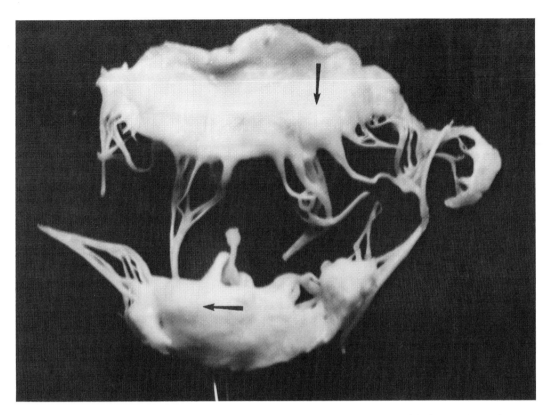

Fig. 2.6. Floppy mitral valve with elongated chordae and interchordal hooding (black arrow). Atrial view.

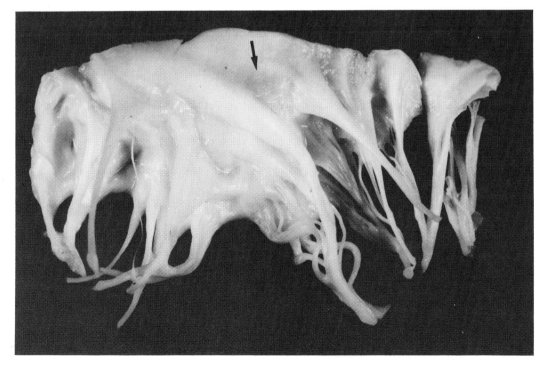

Fig. 2.7. Floppy valve with elongated chordae and interchordal hooding (black arrow). Ventricular view.

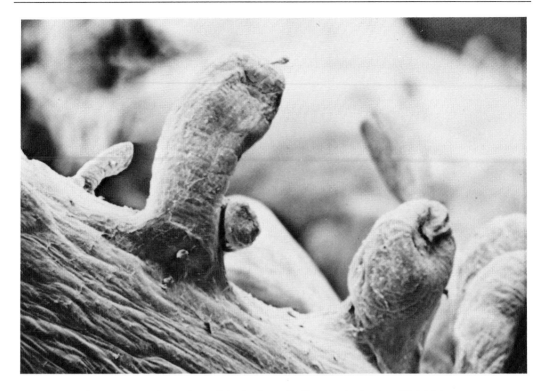

Fig. 2.8. Cystic formations on the surface of the leaflets of a floppy mitral valve. SEM 124x.

tinguished two distinct pathological entities, possibly requiring different surgical approaches. The first was classic myxomatous degeneration with thickened and redundant leaflets (Fig. 2.6 and 2.7), associated with significant annular dilatation and elongation, thickening, and attenuation of main chordae. The second was the so-called fibroelastic deficiency in which leaflets are very thin and not redundant, the annulus is usually only slightly dilated, and chordae are very thin and elongated (Fig. 2.15). Chordal rupture is frequently limited to the posterior leaflet only, mostly to the central portion, and almost always affects first order chordae.[25]

Chordal elongation and posterior leaflet prolapse may result in friction between chordae and endocardium of the posterior ventricular wall producing fibrous alterations of the endocardium that sometimes fuses with the related chordae.[26] Isolated calcifications of these lesions can be seen (Fig. 2.16), independent of the calcifications of mitral annulus reported in some cases of floppy valve.[6,11,27] These areas and the pouches of the posterior leaflet derived from

the adhesion of related chordae to the ventricular endocardial surface may be sources of emboli. Transient ischemic episodes are a feature of floppy mitral syndrome (Fig. 2.17).[26]

Analyzing the changes in mitral insufficiency produced by rheumatic pathology, Barlow[28] stressed the various mechanisms involved in rheumatic chordal modifications. Similar to what is observed in chronic ischemic regurgitation,[29] the predominant factor producing chordal elongation in these cases is increased systolic tensile stress. In fact the primary change observed in active rheumatic carditis, producing pure mitral regurgitation, is dilatation of the posterior annulus.[28] The leaflet area-to-orifice area ratio is altered; this produces a critical reduction of the appositional area between leaflets that in normal hearts is the site of discharge of most of the pressure generated by ventricular contraction. As a result, tension on mitral chordae is markedly increased. They elongate and may finally rupture, producing regurgitation that further aggravates chordal stress, generating a vicious cycle.

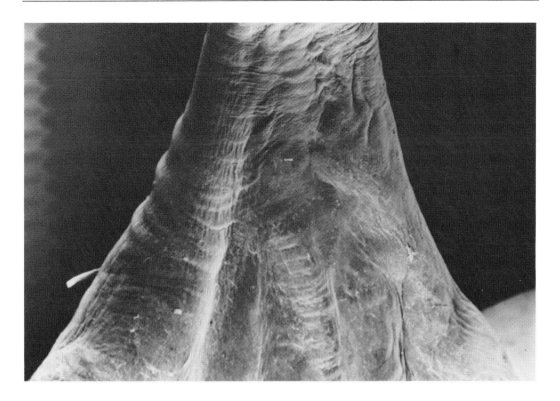

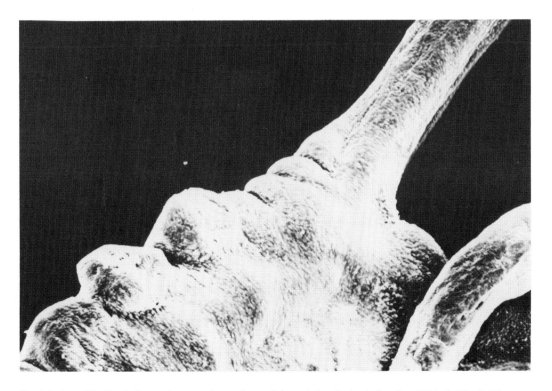

Fig. 2.9 A and B. Cystic formations on the surface of the origin of mitral chordae. SEM, A 50x, B 25x.

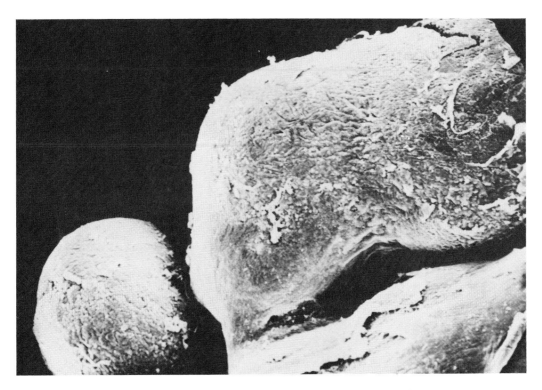

Fig. 2.10. Higher magnification of cystic formations on the surface of mitral chordae. SEM 120x.

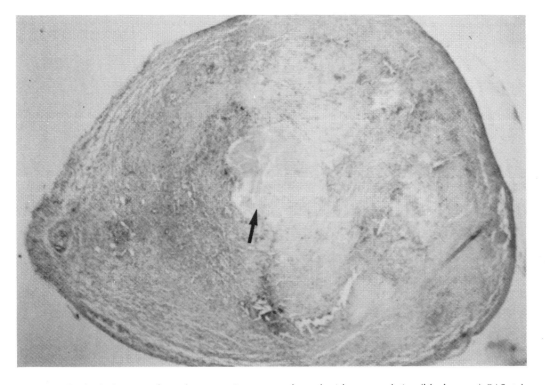

Fig. 2.11. Histological aspect of cyst demonstrating mucopolysaccharide accumulation (black arrow). PAS stain.

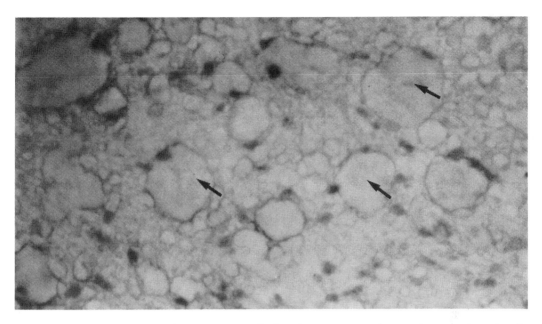

Fig. 2.12. Histological aspect of a myxomatous leaflet showing accumulation of mucopolysaccharides (arrows). H-E stain.

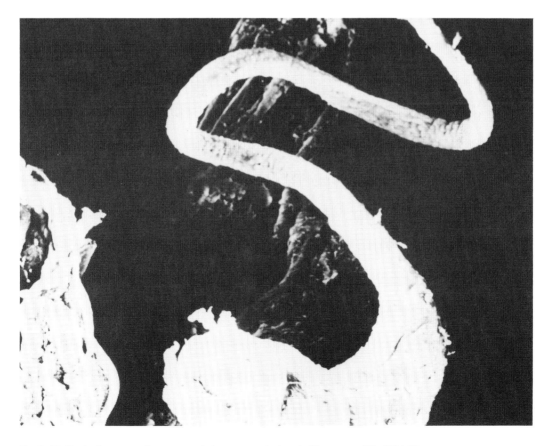

Fig. 2.13. Typical aspect of a ruptured degenerated chorda ("mouse tail"). SEM 85x.

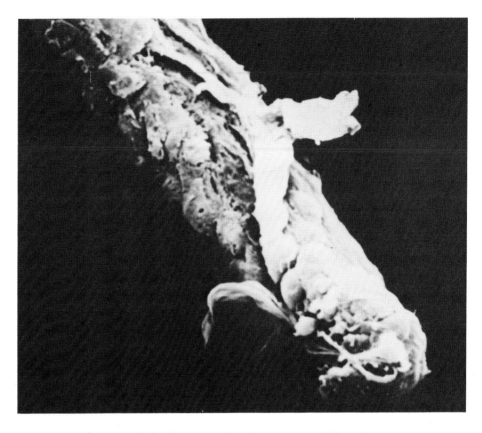

Fig. 2.14. Tip of a ruptured chorda with endothelial damage and fibrin deposition. SEM 630x.

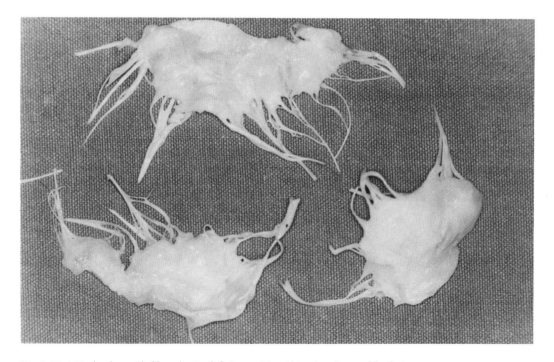

Fig. 2.15. Mitral valve with fibroelastic deficiency. Very thin chordae and leaflets.

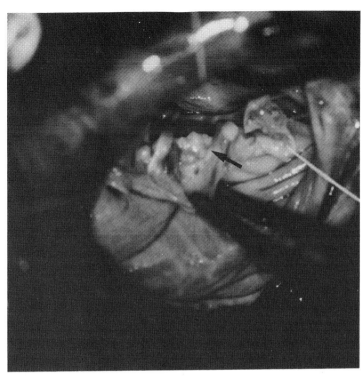

Fig. 2.16. Calcification of the posterior ventricular wall (arrow) corresponding to an area of friction between elongated chordae and the ventricular endocardium.

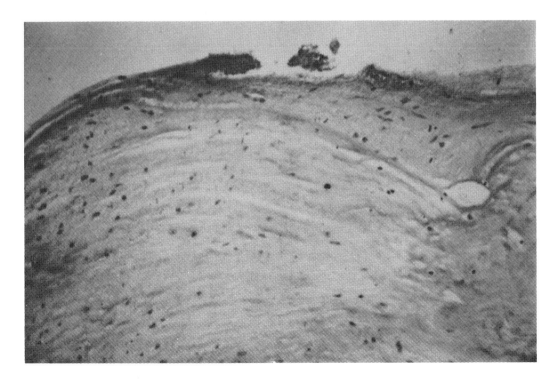

Fig. 2.17. Fibrin deposit corresponding to an endothelial discontinuity of a myxomatous leaflet. Congo red stain.

HISTOLOGY

Unlike the leaflets, which have three layers: the atrialis, the spongiosa, and the fibrosa or ventricularis, normal chordae have only two components: a thick compact fibrous core constituted by tight collagen bundles, fused with the leaflet fibrosa, and a thin external layer of elastic fibers (Figs. 2.18-2.21). In degenerated chordae, observed in cases of floppy mitral valve, the inner fibrous layer has variable areas of collagen tissue infiltration (Figs. 2.22-2.25), disorganization, dissolution, and replacement by acid mucopolysaccharides. Also, elastic fibers fragmentation is frequently observed (Figs. 2.26-2.28).

Hammer[30] reported qualitative changes of valve collagen (absence of type III and type AB collagen) in a case of floppy mitral valve with chordal rupture. On the other hand Cole[31] reported an increased amount of collagen content, mostly type III, interpreting these data as a reparative process in floppy valves, corresponding to the increased cellularity. A possible explanation of the lack of agreement between these two reports may be found in the study by Angelini and co-workers.[32] They found a significant increase of collagen, proteoglycan and elastin in floppy valves, but type III collagen was reduced in valves without fibrosis, while it was increased in valves with evident fibrosis, which is com-

monly observed in the advanced phases of the disease, mostly in the leaflets.[6,12] This histochemical heterogeneity suggests that further research is necessary to clarify the genetic transmission of this disorder since polygenic heritage seems the most probable.[33-35]

The endothelial layer is often affected with surface fissures, fibrin deposition, and subendothelial connective fiber fragmentation (Fig. 2.17). These phenomena probably result from the stress produced by the alteration of cusp geometry and surface tension, related to the underlying degeneration.[36] These quantitative and qualitative changes[19] significantly reduce the resistance to the mechanical stress of valve closure (Fig. 2.29), producing progressive chordal elongation and thinning and the final rupture,[4] that results in flail segments of leaflet tissue.

In rheumatic pathology (Figs. 2.30 and 2.31) fibrous tissue content of the mitral valve is increased, partially replacing normal layers of leaflet and chordae. Chordae are often fused with a compact fibrous core (Fig. 2.32) and a thick external layer with elastic fibers (Fig. 2.33) and fibrous tissue. In floppy valves, cellularity is increased (Figs. 2.34-2.36).

Papillary muscles, chordae, leaflets, and annulus represent a functional unit that coun-

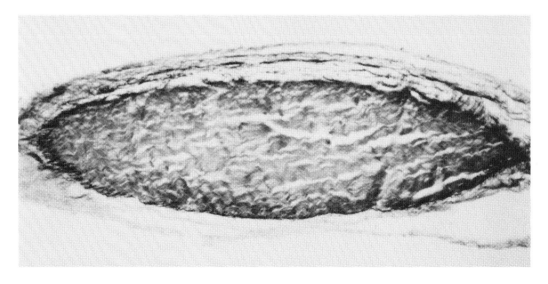

Fig. 2.18. Normal mitral chorda with a thick, compact fibrous core and a thin external layer of elastic fibers. Elastic Weigert-van Gieson stain.

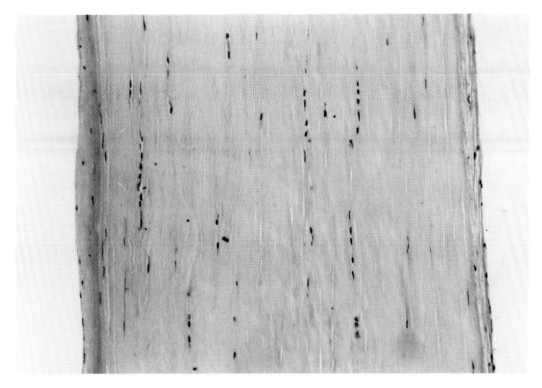

Fig. 2.19. Longitudinal section of a normal chorda. H-E stain.

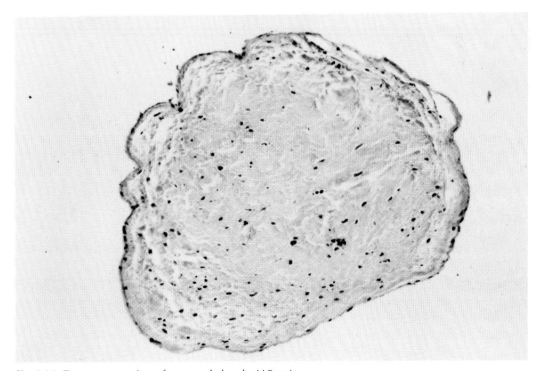

Fig. 2.20. Transverse section of a normal chorda. H-E stain.

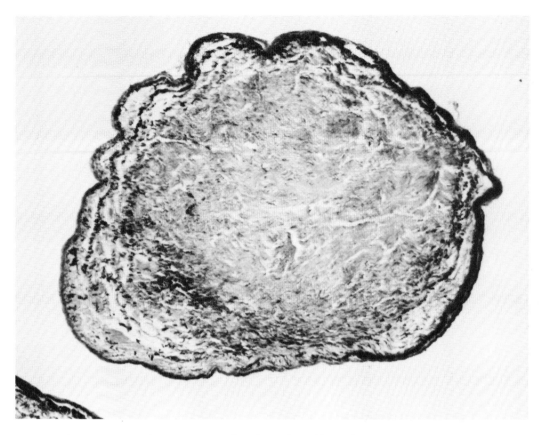

Fig. 2.21. The same section (Fig. 2.20) stained to show elastic fibers. Elastic Weigert-van Gieson stain.

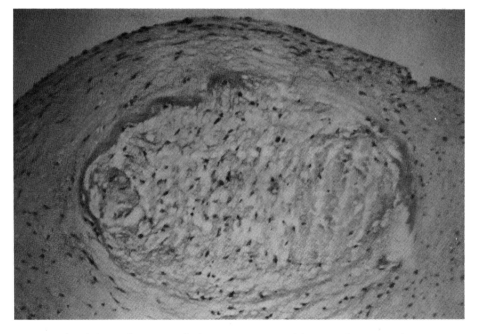

Fig. 2.22. Chorda from a floppy mitral valve. Degeneration of the central core is evident. H-E stain.

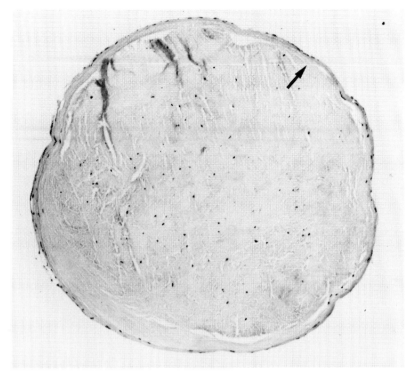

Fig. 2.23. Degenerated chorda. Mucopolysaccharide deposits approximate the endothelial layer (black arrow). H-E stain.

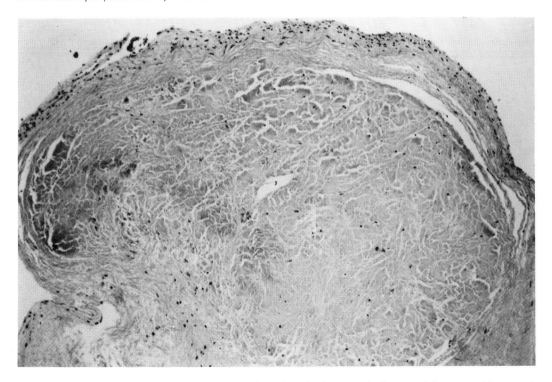

Fig. 2.24. Higher magnification to show mucopolysaccharide deposits, thickening of the external layer and endothelial alterations.

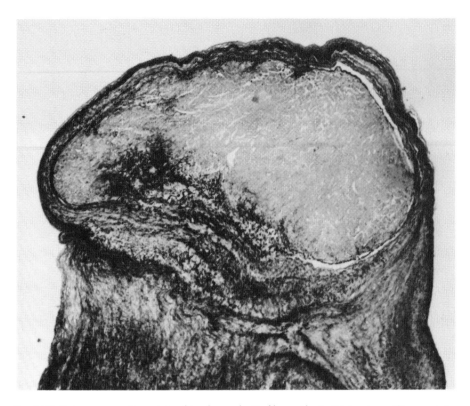

Fig. 2.25. Transverse section stained to show elastic fibers. Elastic Weigert-van Gieson stain.

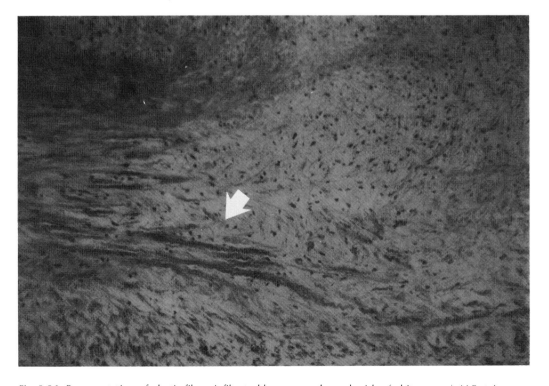

Fig. 2.26. Fragmentation of elastic fibers infiltrated by mucopolysaccharides (white arrow). H-E stain.

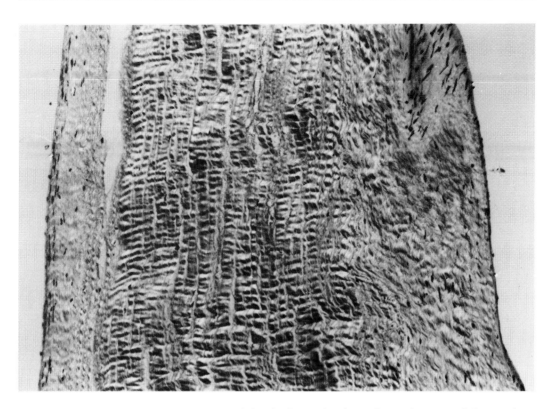

Fig. 2.27. Longitudinal section of a degenerated chorda observed with interferential contrast of phase to show fibers fragmentation and infiltration.

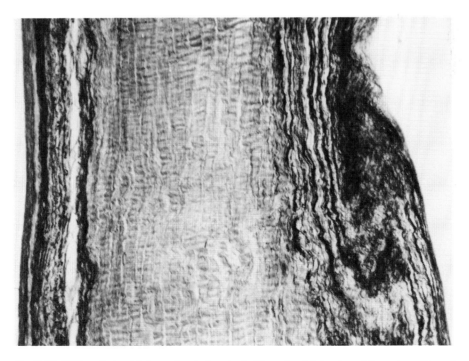

Fig. 2.28. With polarized light and stain for elastic fibers the thickening of the external layer is evident. Elastic Waigert-van Gieson stain.

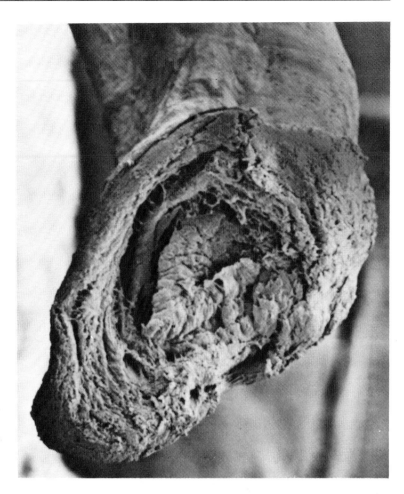

Fig. 2.29. Transverse section of a degenerated chorda showing the myxomatous appearance of the central area, compared with the compact core of normal chordae, which produces a reduction of the resistance to mechanical stress. SEM 85x.

teracts the pressure borne by the leaflets. In cases of leaflet enlargement, as with floppy valve, this balance is compromised, producing increasing traction on the papillary muscles and chordae, and dilatation of the annulus.[37]

The altered distribution of forces, produced by poor apposition of the two leaflets, mostly in cases of chordal rupture, may play a role in increasing myxomatous degeneration.[38] Consistent with this hypothesis is the observation of changes, similar to those observed in floppy valve, in mitral valves replaced for chronic ischemic regurgitation.[29] These specimens have acid mucopolysaccharide deposits in leaflets and chordae with fragmentation and replacement of collagen bundles. Also, in cases of satisfactory valve repair for degenerative mitral incompetence, further chordal rupture is very rare, probably because pressure stress is redistributed among all chordae.[8,20,39]

It is interesting to note that the macroscopic and histological features of floppy mitral valves often involve only segments of the leaflets and some chordae, mostly in the early phase of the disease.

REFERENCES

1. Frater RWM, Ellis Jr FH. The anatomy of canine mitral valve: With notes on function and comparison with other mammalian mitral valves. J Surg Res 1961; 1:171-8.
2. Frater RWM. Mitral valve anatomy and prosthetic valve design. Proceedings staff meeting Mayo Clin 1961; 36:582-92.
3. Anderson RH, Becker AE. Slide atlas of cardiac anatomy. Gower Medical Publishing Ltd, 1980.
4. Baker PB, Bansal GJ, Boudoulas H et al.

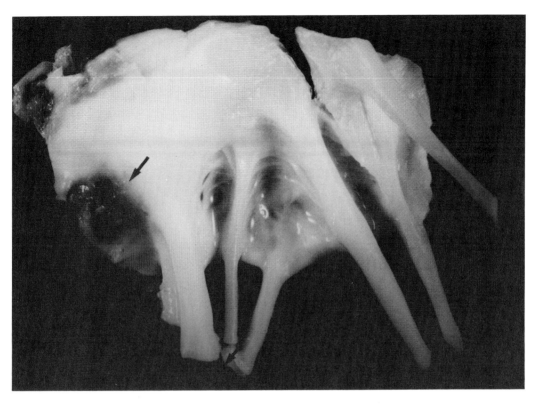

Fig. 2.30. Rheumatic mitral valve with chordal fusion and areas of calcification (arrow).

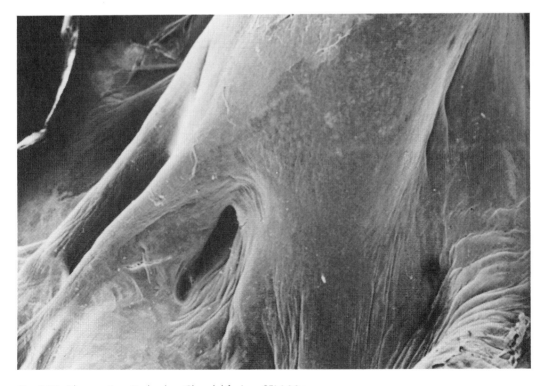

Fig. 2.31. Rheumatic mitral valve. Chordal fusion. SEM 30x.

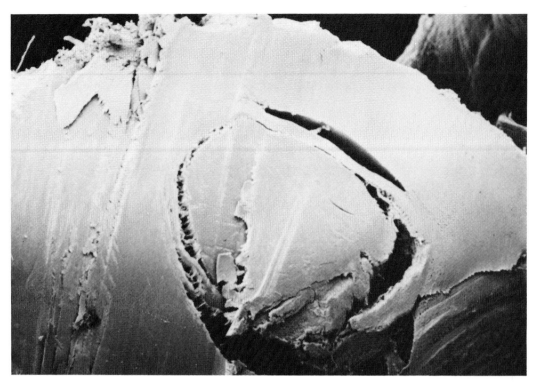

Fig. 2.32. Rheumatic chorda with a compact fibrous core and a thickened external layer. SEM 51x.

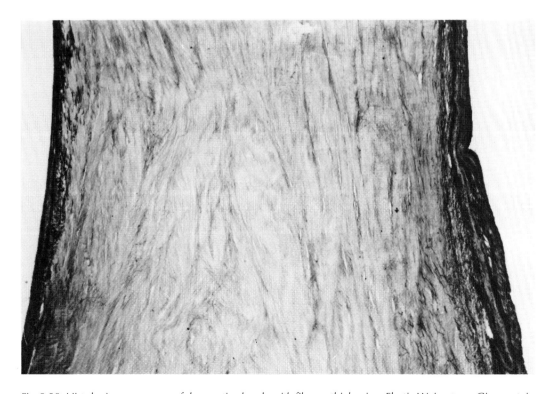

Fig. 2.33. Histologic appearance of rheumatic chorda with fibrous thickening. Elastic Weigert-van Gieson stain.

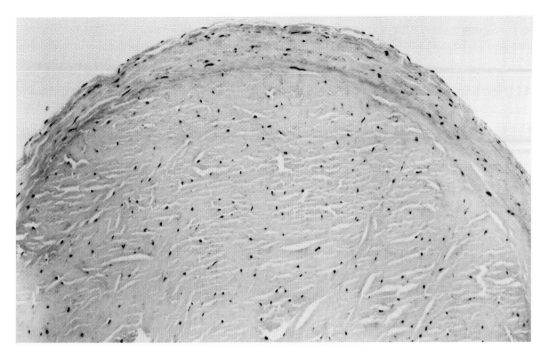

Fig. 2.34. Increased cellularity in the central area of rheumatic chordae, compared with myxomatous chordae.

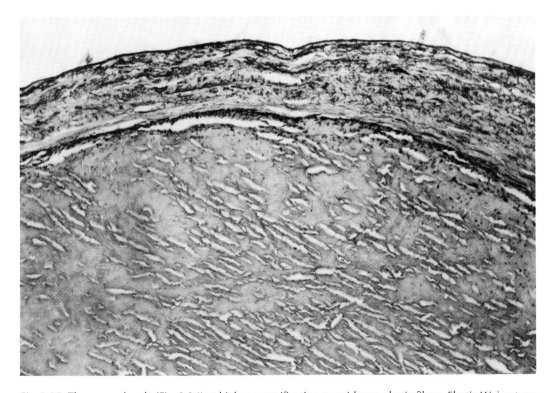

Fig. 2.35. The same chorda (Fig. 2.34) at higher magnification to evidence elastic fibers. Elastic Weigert-van Gieson stain.

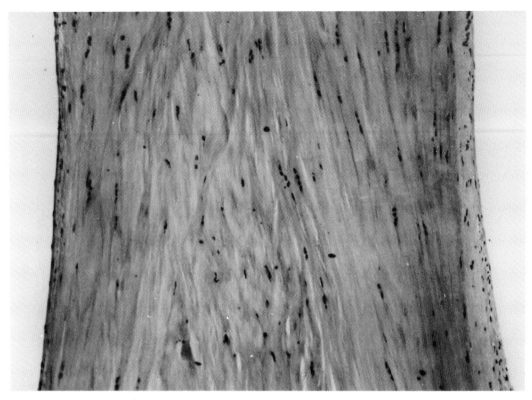

Fig. 2.36. Increased cellularity is seen also in longitudinal section. (See Fig. 2.35) H-E stain.

Floppy mitral valve chordae tendineae: Histopathologic alterations. Hum Pathol 1988; 19:507-12.

5. Frater RWM. Functional anatomy of the mitral valve. In: Ionescu MI, Cohn LH, eds. Mitral valve disease: Diagnosis and treatment. London: Butterworths, 1985:127-38.

6. Titus JL, Edwards JE. Mitral insufficiency other than rheumatic, ischemic, or infective: Emphasis on mitral valve prolapse. Semin Thorac Cardiovasc Surg 1989; 1:118-28.

7. Kunzelman KS, Cochran RP. Mechanical properties of basal and marginal mitral valve chordae tendineae. ASAIO Trans 1990; 36:M 405-8.

8. Frater RWM, Gabbay S, Shore D et al. Reproducible replacement of elongated or ruptured mitral valve chordae. Ann Thorac Surg 1983; 35:14-28.

9. Becker AE, DeWit APM. Mitral valve apparatus. A spectrum of normality relevant to mitral valve prolapse. Br Heart J 1979; 42:680-9.

10. Edwards JE. Pathology of mitral incompe-

tence. In: Silver MD, ed. Cardiovascular Pathology. Vol 1. New York: Churchill Livingstone, 1983:575-98.

11. Wooley CF, Baker PB, Kolibash AJ et al. The floppy, mixomatous mitral valve, mitral valve prolapse, and mitral regurgitation. Prog Cardiovasc Dis 1991; 33:397-433.

12. Hill DG, Davies MJ, Path MC et al. The natural history and surgical management of the redundant cusp syndrome (floppy mitral valve). J Thorac Cardiovasc Surg 1974; 67:519-25.

13. Chandraratna P, Aronow WS. Incidence of ruptured chordae tendineae in mitral valvular prolapse syndrome. Chest 1979; 75:334-9.

14. Grenadier E, Alpan G, Shlomo K et al. The prevalence of ruptured chordae tendineae in mitral valve prolapse syndrome. Am Heart J 1983; 105:603-10.

15. Salomon NW, Stinson EB, Griepp RB et al. Surgical treatment of degenerative mitral regurgitation. Am J Cardiol 1976; 38:463-8.

16. Yacoub M, Halim M, Radley-Smith R et

al. Surgical treatment of mitral regurgitation caused by floppy valves: Repair versus replacement. Circulation 1981; 64 (Suppl II):II 210-II 216.

17. Orszulak TA, Schaff HV, Danielson GK et al. Mitral regurgitation due to ruptured chordae tendineae. J Thorac Cardiovasc Surg 1985; 89:491-8.

18. Kolibash AJ. Progression of mitral regurgitation in patients with mitral valve prolapse. Herz 1988; 13:309-17.

19. Virmani R, Atkinson JB, Forman MB. The pathology of mitral valve prolapse. Herz 1988; 13:215-26.

20. Gregory Jr F, Takeda R, Silva S et al. A new technique for repair of mitral insufficiency caused by ruptured chordae of the anterior leaflet. J Thorac Cardiovasc Surg 1988; 96:765-8.

21. Cosgrove DM. Surgery for degenerative mitral valve disease. Semin Thorac Cardiovasc Surg 1989; 1:183-93.

22. Kolibash AJ, Bush CA, Fontana ME et al. Mitral valve prolapse syndrome: Analysis of 62 patients aged 60 years and older. Am J Cardiol 1983; 52:534-9.

23. Kolibash AJ, Kilman JW, Bush CA et al. Evidence for progression from mild to severe mitral regurgitation in mitral valve prolapse. Am J Cardiol 1986; 58:762-7.

24. Carpentier A, Chauvaud S, Fabiani JN et al. Reconstructive surgery of mitral incompetence. Ten-year appraisal. J Thorac Cardiovasc Surg 1980; 79:338-48.

25. Agozzino L, Thiene G, Valente M et al. Insufficienza mitralica da degenerazione mixoide. Studio patologico di 17 espianti chirurgici. Arch Chir Torac Cardiovasc 1982; 4:85-95.

26. Salazar AE, Edwards JE. Friction lesions of ventricular endocardium. Relation to chordae tendineae of mitral valve. Arch Pathol Lab Med 1970; 90:364-76.

27. Read RC, Thal AP, Wendt VE. Symptomatic valvular myxomatous transformation (the floppy valve syndrome). A possible forme fruste of the Marfan syndrome. Circulation 1965; 32:897-910.

28. Barlow JB. Idiopathic (degenerative) and rheumatic mitral valve prolapse: Historical aspects and an overview. J Heart Valve Dis 1992; 1:163-74.

29. Fishbein MC. Mitral insufficiency in coronary artery disease. Semin Thorac Cardiovasc Surg 1989; 1:129-32.

30. Hammer D, Leier CV, Baba N et al. Altered collagen composition in a prolapsing mitral valve with ruptured chordae tendineae. Am J Med 1979; 67:863-6.

31. Cole WG, Chan D, Hickey AJ et al. Collagen composition of normal and mixomatous human mitral heart valves. Biochem J 1984; 219:451-60.

32. Angelini A, Becker AE, Anderson RH et al. Mitral valve morphology: Normal and mitral valve prolapse. In: Boudoulas H, Wooley CF, eds. Mitral valve prolapse and the mitral valve prolapse syndrome. Mount Kisko, NY: Futura, 1988:13-53.

33. Devereux RB, Kramer-Fox R. Inheritance and phenotypic features of mitral valve prolapse. In: Boudulas H, Wooley CF, eds. Mitral valve prolapse and the mitral valve prolapse syndrome. Mount Kisko, NY: Futura, 1988:109-27.

34. Henney AM, Tsipouras P, Schwartz RC et al. Genetic evidence that mutations in the COL1A1, COL1A2, COL3A1, or COL5A2 collagen genes are not responsible for mitral valve prolapse. Br Heart J 1989; 61:292-9.

35. Wordsworth P, Ogilvie D, Akhras F et al. Genetic segregation analysis of familial mitral valve prolapse shows no linkage to fibrillar collagen genes. Br Heart J 1989; 61:300-6.

36. Pomerance A. Ballooning deformity (mucoid degeneration) of atrioventricular valves. Br Heart J. 1969; 31:343-51.

37. Bryhn M, Garding L. The mitral valve mechanism with normal and prolapsed leaflets in the light of a dynamic model. Clin Cardiol 1986; 9:483-6.

38. Salisbury PF, Cross CE, Rieben PA. Chorda tendinea tension. Am J Physiol 1963; 205:385-92.

39. Duran CG. Surgical management of elongated chordae of the mitral valve. J Cardiac Surg 1989; 4:253-9.

CHAPTER 3

PHYSIOLOGY OF THE SUBVALVULAR APPARATUS

ROLE OF THE CHORDAE TENDINEAE IN MITRAL VALVE MOTION

It is universally accepted that the prevention of valve eversion during systole is not the sole function of the chordae tendinae. Chordal tension throughout diastole was reported by Rushmer,[1] Salisbury,[2] and Padula[3] suggesting an active role during this phase of the cardiac cycle as well. Yet the complete function of these structures is not completely understood.

Computerized simulations and dynamic models have been proposed to assess the components of the mitral apparatus: ventricular wall, papillary muscles, chordae tendineae, valve leaflets, annular ring, and atrial wall.[4-6]

In a series of studies Yellin and co-workers reported the results of acute and chronic animal experiments, patient observation, and computerized models.[4,7-9] These studies focused on the pattern of flow across the mitral valve, and the relative influences of various anatomical and dynamic components. The authors attempted to unify the hypotheses and controversies regarding the mechanisms of mitral valve movements.

The "breaking-jet" theory of Henderson and Johnson[10] affirms that the cusps move to closure before ventricular contraction due to negative pressure on the atrial side of the leaflets produced by the sudden cessation of the blood flow to the ventricles. In 1972 Bellhouse[11] proposed the "vortex-ring" hypothesis that suggests the formation of a vortex system arising from the apex of the ventricular cavity pushing the cusps to closure. Other hypotheses invoke the inversion of the atrioventricular pressure gradient produced by ventricular systole and that of papillary muscle contraction.[12,13]

In a computerized simulation Yellin utilized the equation of motion of the blood-valve-heart system.[4] Introducing the chordae tendineae, under tension throughout diastole, as a force between the ventricular apex and the cusp tip, this simulation described the development of a vortex system pushing the cusps to closure. Their hypothesis holds that there is lateral fluid movement during mitral valve opening and that this force pushes the leaflets beyond their equilibrium position. On the other hand a Venturi effect and the chordae tension draw the cusps together in mid-diastole. This produces shear between blood flow and leaflets creating an expanding vortex also incorporating the "breaking-jet" and driving the valve to closure. It was necessary to invoke chordae under tension during diastole to explain the flow pattern and valve motion during rapid early filling and to produce a vortex system, with the center on the tip of the cusps, that lasts also during atrial contraction.

These findings were also confirmed by an experiment in which the incidental rupture of a papillary muscle produced a grossly regurgitant valve permitting the evaluation of the effect of leaflets partially unsupported by chordae. Consistent with these observations is the recognition that the mitral valve begins to close while the flow is still accelerating.[9] In subsequent studies the authors partially revised their interpretation assuming that deceleration of the flow in mid-diastole coincides with chordae tension to produce the valve movements.[8]

An interesting paper by Binkley and co-workers[14] supported the hypothesis of an active role of papillary muscles and chordae in keeping the leaflets in the equilibrium position during diastole, and determining diastolic valve motions. In patients with spontaneous periods of prolonged atrial and ventricular diastole, they could demonstrate a "semiopen" valve position (52 ±11% of the maximal diastolic opening) maintained despite absent flow, suggesting a role for chordal tension. Indeed in one patient with a Wenckebach rhythm, a case of non-conducted P waves, the authors observed the valve beginning to close early diastole, as with a normal rhythm, and subsequently reopening after a decrease of blood flow to 0 m/s. They concluded that chordae tendineae and papillary muscles play a role in mitral leaflet movements through diastole, confirming the data of Marzilli[13] and Steffens.[15]

The function of both the degree and geometry of chordal tension in leaflet motion was examined by Cape and co-workers.[16] Utilizing in vitro studies to reproduce the displacement of the papillary muscles observed in hypertrophic cardiomyopathy, the authors demonstrated that the systolic anterior motion of the mitral valve, characteristic of this pathology, can be explained by altered distribution and effectiveness of the tethering effect of chordal tension on the leaflets, produced by papillary muscles displacement.

In conclusion the role of the subvalvular apparatus on mitral valve movements is still under investigation, and it will require further studies in order to obtain information that can be applied to surgery. On the other hand the relevance of this apparatus for ventricular function has been known for 30 years.

ROLE OF THE MITRAL SUBVALVULAR APPARATUS IN LEFT VENTRICULAR FUNCTION

In 1964 Lillehei[17] suggested the posterior, and whenever possible the anterior mitral leaflet and chordae be preserved during mitral valve replacement (MVR). The high incidence of low cardiac output syndromes, with a mortality of 37%, after MVR with the excision of leaflets and chordae was related by the author to the change of systolic mechanics of the left ventricle (LV) and the consequent reduction of stroke volume. Previous and subsequent experimental and clinical observations supported this hypothesis.

In 1922 Wiggers[18] described the changing in the LV geometry in different conditions providing the basis for Rushmer's observations regarding the "sphericalization" of the LV.[1,12] This theory suggested that elongation of the short axis and shortening of the long axis produce increased preload of the basal segments of the LV during the isovolumetric phase of systole with an increase in stroke work. The integrity of the subvalvular apparatus is required to demonstrate this event.

A different theory was suggested by Rankin and Olsen[19,20] who demonstrated a relationship between preload and LV geometry during isovolumetric contraction with a spherical shape at small preload volumes and an elliptical shape at larger volumes. However, various causes have been proposed to explain left ventricular dysfunction after mitral valve replacement.

In cases of chronic mitral regurgitation the increase in the afterload produced by the correction of the insufficiency with a prosthesis can decrease function of the myocardium irreversibly damaged by long-standing valve disease.[21,22] Also the current surgical technique for mitral valve replacement, that interrupts papillary muscle-annulus continuity, may influence ventricular performance.

To test this hypothesis Spence and co-workers[23] performed a series of experiments assessing the separate effects produced by the rigid prosthetic ring and by the interruption of the papillary muscles-mitral annulus continuity caused by chordal division. While fixation of the mitral annulus with a standard Bjork-Shiley prosthesis produced a small, insignificant decrease in ventriclular systolic performance (expressed as systolic and developed pressures and dP/dt), division of the chordae tendineae markedly impaired ventricular systolic function, leaving the ventricular compliance (diastolic pressure/diastolic volume) unchanged.

These results confirm the data reported previously by the same group regarding the value of chordae tendineae preservation during mitral valve replacement in experimental and clinical studies.[24,25] The authors proposed an explanation for these observations endorsing Rushmer's theory of ventricular "sphericalization"[1,12,26] with the consequent increase in preload of the circumferential fibers via Starling's law. Moreover they suggested a role for papillary muscle-annulus continuity in reducing the afterload of the basal fibers of the ventricular myocardium, supporting them during contraction, and resulting in enhanced minor axis shortening.

An important contribution to understanding the influence of the subvalvular apparatus on ventricular systolic function was made by the Stanford group. They started their research from the discordant results reported by David[25,27] and Lessana.[28] The former author demonstrated significant deterioration of systolic function after conventional mitral valve replacement despite chordae-sparing procedures (valve repair and valve replacement with preservation of the posterior leaflet and chordae). On the other hand Lessana reported a significant reduction of the ejection fraction after valve repair for chronic regurgitation.

In a canine model Hansen and co-workers[29] studied the perfused in situ LV after dividing all the anterior and posterior chordae. They evaluated the variations of a load-independent parameter, the slope of the peak isovolumetric pressure-volume relationship (Emax).[30] Under controlled conditions Emax decreased from a mean value of 11.97+/-3.35 to 6.38+/-0.96 mm Hg/ml (p<.001) after chordae division. Also dP/dt was affected in the same way and the phenomena were more evident at the larger volume as result of a significant reduction in ventricular elastance. The modifications of the time-varying LV elastance curves during systole, produced by chordal division demonstrated that the positive influence of the subvalvular apparatus on this parameter extends throughout cardiac cycle. Significant changes in the shape of the ventricular cavity were recorded by fluoroscopy. The areas of insertion of the papillary muscles contract uniformly with the other sectors of the ventricle during the isovolumetric phase of systole in the presence of an intact subvalvular apparatus, while they bulge after chordal division and move dyskinetically. The authors suggested two hypotheses to explain their results. First a positive "feedback system" resulting in the transmission of the upward forces, pushing the mitral leaflets during systole to the areas of insertion of the papillary muscles along intact chordae and increasing the force generated by these areas. A second possible explanation holds that the subvalvular apparatus "tethers" the ventricle maintaining the optimum geometric configuration throughout systole.

In another paper the same authors[31] reported the results of research on the relative contributions of anterior and posterior chordae (divided consecutively) to ventricular systolic function in a canine model. Analyzing the variations of Emax, they found that the difference between the relative contributions to Emax of anterior versus posterior chordae was not statistically significant, although anterior chordae seem to play a major role. Moreover they could not find any influence related to the order of chordae divided. Indeed the value of Emax decreased by 27% when anterior chordae alone were divided and by an additional 16% when posterior chordae were subsequently cut. With the reverse order of division the reductions were 17% (posterior chordae) and 24% (anterior chordae), respectively. The combined contribution of the chordae to peak left ventricular elastance ranged from 41% to 43% while the balance, 57-59%,could be attributed to the ventricular myocardium, that in the past had been considered the only component influencing LV pump function.

The significance of the posterior component of papillary muscle-annulus continuity (posterior annular chordae) in maintaining the efficacy of LV wall motion had been previously stressed by Rushmer,[1] and Hagl et al.[3] Also Sarris et al[33] evaluated the effect of chordae reattachment on Emax. In a swine model, they observed a significant reduction of Emax with the detachment of all chordae and complete restoration of ventricular function after reattachment with a statistically insignificant difference between baseline and final values of Emax. It is important to note that all experiments performed by this group involved sham-operated animal controls in order to exclude a time-related deterioration of the model and the considerable influence of anesthesia and surgical technique on the results. The authors claim that the absence of sham controls by Spence et al[34] could explain why they were unable to demonstrate improvement in ventricular performance after reattachment of a previously divided papillary muscle.

Contradictory results have been reported as well by Salter and co-workers.[35] They measured the contribution of the subvalvular apparatus to LV function utilizing intracavitary pressure catheters and piezoelectric sonomicrometry crystals to determine wall thickness, major-axis and minor-axis of the ventricle. After removing the native valve with all chordae, they anchored a 3-0 monofilament suture to the head of each papillary muscle, exteriorizing these artificial chordae in paravalvular position, so that they could maintain the papillary muscles in "attached" and "detached" states. A bileaflet mechanical prosthesis was then implanted. While they observed significant differences in major-axis end-diastolic length (66.9 ±1.7 mm at control versus 69.9 ±1.9 mm in detached state), in peak systolic left ventricular pressure and peak dP/dt that were

lower in attached state, all other load-dependent and -independent changes were statistically insignificant. With these findings the authors were unable to confirm the hypothesis that the interruption of valvular-ventricular continuity, by severing mitral chordae, produces an impairment in LV systolic function. However the same authors emphasized that these results were obtained in normal canine hearts, in acute experiments that could be extrapolated to patients with chronically dilated or hypertrophic left ventricles only with difficulty. Also discussing the contradiction between these data and those from their own experiments, Sarris et al[33] observed that the accuracy of artificial chordae tension was not controlled in Salter et al's preparations and, moreover, the "attached" state may have been inadequate to reproduce the distribution of forces between annulus and ventricular wall, since only one chorda anchored each papillary muscle to one point on the annulus. This is consistent with the old report by Salisbury and co-workers,[2] who observed that tension in one chorda increases when all other chordae are severed, suggesting a distribution of the total tension, generated between mitral annulus and ventricular wall, among all chordae.

Since experiments based on evaluation of load-independent parameters irrefutably demonstrated the influence of valvular-ventricular interaction on global LV systolic function,[43] the Stanford group performed other animal studies[37-39] to evaluate the relevance of the subvalvular apparatus for LV regional mechanics. Canine and swine models were utilized with both in situ isovolumetric and ejecting hearts.

In the first series of animals (isovolumetric swine preparations) they examined a compliant intraventricular balloon filled with radiographic contrast, before and after severing all chordae. The experiments demonstrated significant decline in global LV systolic function, with a major decrease in elastance in the area of insertion of the posteromedial papillary muscle, while the end-diastolic pressure-volume relationship was unchanged. This indicated that during diastole LV function was unchanged after chordae detachment. Also three-dimensional contraction synergy was significantly decreased. The greatest effects occurred when the origin of the polar coordinate was loctated in the apical aspect of the long-axis of the left ventricular.

Gams and co-workers[40-42] assessed the influence of the subvalvular apparatus on left ventricular dimensions and function in canine ejecting preparations. They performed mitral valve replacement leaving in place the entire mitral apparatus; then ventricular function was evaluated before and after chordal division (by exteriorized wires). There was a sudden shift in opposite directions of the pressure-length relationship between the two axes, although of different degree. Indeed there is a significant increase in LV end-diastolic volume (18%) and end-diastolic major-axis length (10%) associated with reduced systolic shortening (20% to 43%) at all preload values, while a less significant decrease in end-diastolic length of the minor-axis and increased systolic shortening, significant only at low end-diastolic pressure values, were observed. These changes were more remarkable if intracavitary diameters measurements are considered. The interruption of the subvalvular apparatus caused impairment of LV systolic function, expressed as a significant decrease of dP/dt-max (by 9-15%), ejection fraction (16%) and stroke volume (up to 24%).

After their experiments in isovolumetric hearts, Sarris and co-workers[37] also confirmed the role of the mitral apparatus in global and regional systolic function in ejecting canine preparations. A significant decrease in global function was demonstrated by load-dependent and load-independent parameters. Impairment of systolic function was not uniform. Greater variations were observed in the anteroposterior minor-axis, and was unaffected again.

Clinical evidence for the role of papillary muscle-annulus continuity on LV systolic function was reported by Corin and co-workers.[43] A significant difference in several parameters analyzing LV systolic function was observed between patients who had undergone mitral valve repair (MVR) and those with MVR without preservation of the subvalvular apparatus. Systolic dysfunction was particularly evident in the areas of papillary muscle insertion.

The question of the role of the subvalvular apparatus on LV diastolic function was addressed by Dyke and co-workers.[44] Analyzing the effects of papillary-annular discontinuity after MVR on LV diastolic properties, they found a significant increase of the isovolumetric time constant and LV end-diastolic minor axis length only in overloaded canine hearts, while no differences were found in normally loaded preparations. Alterations in myocardial stiffness were absent in both groups. Changes of the active component of diastole may be related to the modified LV geometry produced by chordal interruption.

To separate the effects of anterolateral and posteromedial papillary muscle chordae on ventricular function, Yun and co-workers[39] evaluated the consequences of randomly severing one group of chordae, followed by division of the other group, in canine ejecting hearts. Systolic function declined in the regions of insertion of papillary muscles as well as in free wall areas far from them. No differences were observed with regard to the order of chordal division. Moreover, the effect of anterolateral chordae was more pronounced in areas of papillary muscle insertion, while both groups of chordae influenced contractility of remote free wall areas without significant difference.

The influence of the subvalvular apparatus after MVR was analyzed in open-chest ejecting canine hearts, before and after chordal division with exteriorized snares, by the same group of authors.[45] The variations of curvilinear end-systolic pressure-volume relationship (ESPVR), end-systolic volume at 100 mmHg end-systolic pressure (V100), preload recruitable stroke work (SW) and end-diastolic volume (EDV) at SW of 1,000 mmHg.ml (Vw1,000) demonstrated a deterioration of global LV systolic function after chordal division. In fact the coefficient of nonlinearity of ESPVR was less negative by 90%, the slope of ESPVR at the volume axis intercept decreased by 75%, V100 by 42%, SW by 14%, while Vw1,000 increased by 17%. Moreover the mechanical energy generated by the LV significantly decreased (decrease of the slope of the pressure volume area-EDV relationship). Also the efficiency of converting mechanical energy into external work was equally reduced by 14%. Analyzing ventriculo-arterial coupling,[46-47] expressed as a ratio between systemic arterial elastance (Ea) and the slope of the linear ESPVR (Ees), the authors observed a significant increase of this indicator (Ea/Ees = 1 for maximal external output) due to a decrease of Ea associated with a greater decline of Ees.

In a recent study in patients with longstanding mitral regurgitation, Starling[48] demonstrated that the mechanical efficiency of LV stroke work is maintained by the low energy requirement for the regurgitant jet, with regard to myocardial dysfunction occurs. On the contrary, energy transfer to the arterial system is depressed. The author[49] reported the normalization of LV-arterial coupling with significant increase in transfer of energy from the LV to the arterial system, after correction of chronic mitral regurgitation.

The clinically very relevant question if data obtained from "normal acute" isovolumetric or ejecting preparations could be properly compared to findings involving "chronically diseased" hearts was addressed by Yun and co-workers.[50] After producing mitral regurgitation in dogs, without injury to the subvalvular apparatus, and after consequent chronic left ventricular dilatation, MVR was performed preserving mitral chordae. Left ventricular function was evaluated before and after dividing all chordae. Utilizing loaddependent and -independent parameters, a significant decrease in global ventricular systolic function was observed after chordal division. Moreover increased global and regional afterload (increased wall stress) and reduced external stroke work were produced by chordal division. A significant mismatch was confirmed in ventriculo-arterial coupling, expression of the interaction between LV function and systemic circulation elastance. It was produced by a decrease in ventricular efficiency associated with increased afterload and reduction of ventricular preload reserve.

Similarly, observations on chronically diseased hearts were reported by Pitarys et[51] in a clinical study. After a mean interval of more than 10 years after valve replacement, 21 patients underwent cardiac catheterization for suspected prosthesis dysfunction. They confirmed regional left ventricular dysfunction after traditional MVR, with excision of the subvalvular apparatus. The ejection fraction and the average radial shortening were not significantly changed compared with the pre-operative hemodynamics, while significant decrease in radial shortening in the area of posteromedial papillary muscle insertion was observed. The authors could not demonstrate similar evidence for the antero-lateral papillary muscle insertion area because this region was not adequately visualized in the angiograms. Based on these observations, they suggested the presence of adaptive mechanisms to improve left ventricular function after the contribution of the subvalvular apparatus has been withdrawn by valve replacement. These phenomena take place over a long period since studies performed soon after the operation revealed significant reduction of LV systolic performance.[27-28,52-54] Additionally, these mechanisms don't compensate completely for changes produced by chordal division as long as significant areas of hypokinesia persist for several years after mitral valve replacement.[51]

A positive segmental effect on LV systolic function after mitral repair, compared with MVR, was reported by Sakai et al.[55] Eight months after surgery they found global ejection fraction unchanged in patients who had undergone repair, while this parameter was decreased after MVR. This was mainly related to a significant reduction of the ejection fraction at the level of the subannular area, after MVR, while it was maintained after repair.

Rozich et al[56] also investigated postoperative LV ejection performance after MVR and mitral repair. Although the so-called "low-impedance regurgitant jet"[21,57-58] was abolished with both procedures, LV ejection was reduced only after MVR. Analyzing two groups of patients one week after MVR or mitral repair they found a significant increase in LV end-systolic stress after MVR, while this index was reduced after repair. Also LV fractional shortening decreased after MVR, while it was unchanged after repair. All parameters (enddiastolic dimension, end-systolic dimension, end-systolic stress, and fractional shortening) were more favorable after repair than after MVR, indicating that maintaining LV size and geometry after repair reduces end-systolic stress and preserves LV ejection performance, counterbalancing the abolition of the "low-impedance regurgitant jet."

In 1969 Braunwald[59] suggested an explanation for reduction of LV wall stress in mitral insufficiency. The incompetence of the valve allows the shortening of myocardial fibers to start at the onset of systole, removing the isovolumetric phase of LV systole. This mechanism produces, in turn, reduction of the radius of the LV cavity and decreased wall stress.[60]

The influence of LV geometry on the decline of ejection fraction observed after correction of chronic mitral regurgitation was also recently analyzed by Goldfine and co-workers.[61] In patients with preserved preoperative LV systolic function, they found that wall stress (afterload) was not significantly modified with postoperative reduction of LV size, while ejection fraction significantly fell in all cases. This suggests a role for decreased preload and elimination of the subvalvular apparatus, with consequent abnormal long axis shortening, in decreasing postoperative ejection fraction.

Similar deterioration of LV function after MVR for chronic mitral regurgitation was reported by Peter[52] and Phillips.[53] In patients with ventricles already impaired by longstanding valve insufficiency, sudden increase in LV afterload, produced by obliteration of the regurgitant jet, may significantly contribute to this deterioration.

Acute increase in LV afterload associated with correction of mitral regurgitation had been suggested, in fact, by Spratt and co-workers.[62] In a conscious canine model they evaluated the effect of closure of a shunt created from the LV to the left atrium. Forward stroke volume, wall stress, peak pressure and ventricular efficiency increased, while LV fractional shortening and total stroke volume decreased. In other words, LV pump function, defined as forward output at comparable filling pressure, improves, although global ejection fraction is impaired

by acute increase in afterload. Similar data documenting an increase in afterload after MVR in cases of mitral regurgitation were reported by Harpole and co-workers in clinical setting.[63]

Different conclusions have been presented in a recent paper by Gaasch and Zile.[64] They evaluated ventricular systolic wall stress (afterload) before and after MVR for chronic mitral regurgitation to confirm the generally believed afterload reduction effect produced by the "low-impedance regurgitant flow" into the left atrium, as well as to evaluate the relationship between decrease in LV ejection fraction and elimination of the regurgitant flow, produced by MVR.[65] Before operation, the authors recorded normal or high ventricular wall stress indicating no afterload reduction produced by the regurgitant jet.

A different response was observed in patients who underwent MVR in decompensated versus compensated status. In the former group afterload increased, with a possibly related reduction of the ejection fraction; on the other hand, in the latter group presented wall stress was reduced, although a concomitant decline of fiber shortening was present. These data suggest again the significant effect of the discontinuation of papillary-leaflet-annulus continuity on postoperative ventricular performance rather than on increased afterload.

In surgical procedures for mitral stenosis, such as commissurotomy, preservation of the subvalvular apparatus improves ventricular function when compared with traditional MVR without preservation of the subvalvular apparatus. In two groups of patients who underwent MVR or mitral commissurotomy, respectively, postoperative end-diastolic volume, stroke volume, and ejection fraction were analyzed by Kazama et al.[66] All parameters increased in both groups. Yet regional systolic wall motion improved only after commissurotomy; it declined after MVR.

In conclusion the subvalvular apparatus (papillary muscles and chordae tendineae) irrefutably plays asubstantial role in LV function throughout the cardiac cycle. During diastole this consists mainly in reinforcing blood flow forces to produce mitral leaflet movements and positions and to maintain the optimum LV geometry compatible with a chronically diseased heart. During systole the functions are more complex and still not completely understood.[67] Besides prevention of valve eversion and support for leaflet apposition to prevent valve regurgitation, chordae and papillary muscles significantly enhance LV systolic function. Mechanisms suggested to explain this role can be summarized as follows:

Papillary muscles and chordae improve systolic function by maintaining the optimal configuration of the ventricular cavity throughout systole by tethering the mitral valve to the ventricular wall. This mechanism may produce a local preload increase of the circumferential fibers in the basal segments of the ventricle, and, more effectively, may reduce the regional afterload. The latter effect has important clinical consequences in patients with dilated ventricles due to chronic mitral regurgitation in which surgical correction may produce a significant increase in ventricular afterload by the abolition of low-impedance regurgitant flow. Therefore interruption of the valve-ventricular continuity increases wall tension in order to maintain the stroke work. Preload increases and ventricular efficiency declines significantly.

The clinical implications of the preservation of the subvalvular apparatus in mitral valve replacement will be discussed in Chapter 10.

REFERENCES

1. Rushmer RF, Finlayson BL, Nash AA. Movements of the mitral valve. Circ Res 1956; 4:337-42.
2. Salisbury PF, Cross CE, Rieben PA. Chorda tendinea tension. Am J Physiol 1963; 205:385-92.
3. Padula RT, Cowan GSM, Camishion RC. Photographic analysis of the active and passive components of cardiac valvular action. J Thorac Cardiovasc Surg 1968; 56:790-8.
4. Yellin EL, Peskin CS, Frater RWM. Pulsatile flow across the mitral valve: Hydraulic, electronic and digital computer simulation. ASME, Proceedings Winter Annual Meeting, New York, November 26-30, 1972, No. 72 WA/BHF-10.
5. Bryhn M, Garding L. The mitral valve mechanism with normal and prolapsed leaflets in the light of a dynamic model. Clin Cardiol 1986; 9:483-6.
6. Miller GE, Marcotte H. Computer simulation of human mitral valve mechanics and motion. Comput Biol Med 1987; 17:305-19.
7. Yellin E, Peskin C, Yoran C et al. Mechanisms of mitral valve motion during diastole. Am J Physiol 1981; 241 (Heart Circ Physiol):H 389-H 400.
8. Karen G, Meissner JS, Sherez J et al. Interrelationship of mid-diastolic mitral valve motion, pulmonary venous flow, and transmitral flow. Circulation 1986; 74:36-44.
9. Yellin EL, Yoran C, Frater RWM. Physiology of mitral valve flow. In: Duran C, Angell WW, Johnson AD, Oury JH, eds. Recent progress in mitral valve disease. London: Butterworths, 1984:47-59.
10. Henderson Y, Johnson E. Two modes of closure of the heart valves. Heart 1912; 4:69-82.
11. Bellhouse BJ. Fluid mechanics of a model mitral valve and left ventricle. Cardiovasc Res 1972; 6:199-210.
12. Rushmer R. Initial phase of ventricular systole: Asynchronous contraction. Am J Physiol 1956; 188:187-94.
13. Marzilli M, Sabbah HN, Lee T et al. Role of the papillary muscle in opening and closure of the mitral valve. Am J Physiol 1980; 238 (Heart Circ Physiol):H 348-H 354.
14. Binkley PF, Bonagura JD, Olson SM et al. The equilibrium position of the mitral valve: An accurate model of mitral valve motion in humans. Am J Cardiol 1987; 59:109-13.
15. Steffens T, Hagan A. Role of chordae tendineae in mitral valve opening: Two-dimensional echcardiographic evidence. Am J Cardiol 1984; 53:153-6.
16. Cape EG, Simons D, Jimoh A et al. Chordal geometry determines the shape and extent of systolic anterior mitral motion: In vitro studies. J Am Coll Cardiol 1989; 13:1438-48.
17. Lillehei CW, Levy MJ, Bonnabeau RC. Mitral valve replacement with preservation of the papillary muscles and the chordae tendineae. J Thorac Cardiovasc Surg 1964; 47:532-43.

18. Wiggers CJ, Katz LN. The contour of the ventricular volume curves under different conditions. Am J Physiol 1922; 58:439-75.

19. Rankin JS, McHale PA, Arentzen CE et al. The three-dimensional dynamic geometry of the left ventricle in the conscious dog. Circ Res 1976; 39:304-13.

20. Olsen CO, Rankin JS, Arentzen CE et al. The deformational characteristics of the left ventricle in the conscious dog. Circ Res 1981; 49:843-55.

21. Rankin JS, Nicholas LM, Kouchoukos NT. Experimental mitral regurgitation: Effects on left ventricular function before and after elimination of chronic regurgitation in the dog. J Thorac Cardiovasc Surg 1975; 70:478-88.

22. Rapaport E. Natural history of aortic and mitral valve disease. Am J Cardiol 1975; 35:221-7.

23. Spence PA, Peniston CM, David TE et al. Toward a better understanding of the etiology of left ventricular dysfunction after mitral valve replacement: An experimental study with possible clinical implications. Ann Thorac Surg 1986; 41:363-71.

24. David TE, Strauss AD, Mesher E et al. Is it important to preserve the chordae tendineae and papillary muscles during mitral valve replacement? Can J Surg 1981; 24:236-9.

25. David TE, Burns RJ, Bacchus CM et al. Mitral valve replacement for mitral regurgitation with and without preservation of chordae tendineae. J Thorac Cardiovasc Surg 1984; 88:718-25.

26. Rushmer RF. Cardiovascular dynamics. Philadelphia: Saunders, 1970.

27. David TE, Uden DE, Strauss HD. The importance of the mitral apparatus in left ventricular function after correction of mitral regurgitation. Circulation 1983; 68 (Suppl II):II 76-II 82.

28. Lessana A, Herreman F, Boffety C et al. Hemodynamic and cineangiographic study before and after mitral valvuloplasty (Carpentier's technique). Circulation 1981; 64 (Suppl II): II 195.

29. Hansen DE, Cahill PD, DeCampli WM et al. Valvular-ventricular interaction: Importance of the mitral apparatus in canine left ventricular systolic performance. Circulation 1986; 73:1310-20.

30. Suga H, Sagawa K, Shoukas AA. Load independence of the instantaneous pressure-volume ratio of the left ventricle and effect of epinephrine and heart rate on the ratio. Circ Res 1973; 32:314-22.

31. Hansen DE, Cahill PD, Derby GC et al. Relative contributions of the anterior and posterior mitral chordae tendineae to canine global left ventricular systolic performance. J Thorac Cardiovasc Surg 1987; 93:45-55.

32. Hagl S, Heimisch H, Meisner H et al. In-situ function of the papillary muscles in the intact canine left ventricle. In: Duran C, Angell WW, Johnson AD, Oury JH, eds. Recent progress in mitral valve disease. London: Butterworths, 1984:397-409.

33. Sarris GE, Cahill PD, Hansen DE et al. Restoration of left ventricular systolic performance after reattachment of the mitral chordae tendineae: The importance of valvular-ventricular interaction. J Thorac Cardiovasc Surg 1988; 95:969-79.

34. Spence PA, Peniston CM, Mihic N et al. A physiological approach to surgery for acute rupture of the papillary muscle. Ann Thorac Surg 1986; 42:27-30.

35. Salter DR, Pellom GL, Murphy CE et al. Papillary-annular continuity and left ventricular systolic function after mitral valve replacement. Circulation 1986; 74 (Suppl I): I 121-I 129.

36. Sarris GE, Miller DC. Valvular-ventricular interaction: The importance of the mitral chordae tendineae in terms of global left ventricular systolic function. J Cardiac Surg 1988; 3:215-34.

37. Sarris GE, Fann JI, Niczyporuk MA et al. Global and regional left ventricular systolic performance in the in-situ ejecting canine heart: Importance of the mitral apparatus. Circulation 1989; 80 (Suppl I):I 24-I 42.

38. Hansn DE, Sarris GE, Niczyporuk MA et al. Physiologic role of the mitral apparatus in left ventricular regional mechanics, contraction synergy, and global systolic performance. J Thorac Cardiovasc Surg 1989; 97:521-33.

39. Yun KL, Fann JI, Rayhill SC et al. Importance of the mitral subvalvular apparatus for left ventricular segmental systolic me-

chanics. Circulation 1990; 82 (Suppl IV): IV 89-IV 104.

40. Gams E, Schad H, Heimisch W et al. Preservation versus severance of the subvalvular apparatus in mitral valve replacement: An experimental study. Eur J Cardio-thorac Surg 1990; 4:250-6.

41. Gams E, Hagl S, Schad H et al. Significance of the subvalvular apparatus for left-ventricular dimensions and systolic function: Experimental replacement of the mitral valve. Thorac Cardiovasc Surgeon 1991; 39:5-12.

42. Gams E, Hagl S, Schad H et al. Importance of the mitral apparatus for left ventricular function: An experimental approach. Eur J Cardio-thorac Surg 1992; 6 (Suppl 1):S17-S24.

43. Corin WJ, Hess OM, Krogmann ON et al. Regional wall motion after surgery for chronic mitral regurgitation: Valve reconstruction vs replacement. Circulation 1992; 86 (Suppl I):I 539.

44. Dyke CM, Lutz HA, Brunsting LA et al. Diastolic function after mitral valve replacement. Circulation 1990; 82 (Suppl III):III 480.

45. Yun KL, Niczyporuk MA, Sarris GE et al. Importance of mitral subvalvular apparatus in terms of cardiac energetics and systolic mechanics in the ejecting canine heart. J Clin Invest 1991; 87:247-54.

46. Asanoi H, Sasayama S, Kameyama T. Ventriculoarterial coupling in normal and failing heart in humans. Circ Res 1989; 65:483-93.

47. Burkhoff D, Sagawa K. Ventricular efficiency predicted by an analytical model. Am J Physiol 1986; 73:161-71.

48. Starling MR. Mechanical efficiency of performing volume work in long-term mitral regurgitation. Circulation 1992; 86 (Suppl I):I 459.

49. Starling MR. Effects of valve surgery for long-term mitral regurgitation on left ventricular-arterial coupling relations. Circulation 1992; 86 (Suppl I):I 540.

50. Yun KL, Rayhill SC, Niczyporuk MA et al. Mitral valve replacement in dilated canine hearts with chronic mitral regurgitation. Importance of the mitral subvalvular apparatus. Circulation 1991; 84 (Suppl III): III 112-III 124.

51. Pitaris CJ II, Forman MB, Panayiotou H et al. Long-term effects of excision of the mitral apparatus on global and regional ventricular function in humans. J Am Coll Cardiol 1990; 15:557-63.

52. Peter CA, Austin EH, Jones RH. Effect of valve replacement for chronic mitral insufficiency on left ventricular function during rest and exercise. J Thorac Cardiovasc Surg 1981; 82:127-35.

53. Phillips HR, Levine FH, Carter JE et al. Mitral valve replacement for isolated mitral regurgitation: Analysis of clinical course and late postoperative left ventricular ejection fraction. Am J Cardiol 1981; 48:647-54.

54. Huysmans H. Mitral valve structure and function: Considerations for repair and replacement. In: Proceedings Medtronic Cardiovascular Technology Symposium. Ayrshire, Scotland, 1991.

55. Sakai K, Sakaki S, Hirata N et al. Assessment of postoperative left ventricular function after mitral valve repair for mitral regurgitation. Circulation 1991; 84 (Suppl II):II 578.

56. Rozich J, Carabello B, Usher B et al. A mechanism by which ejection performance is preserved following mitral valve repair but not replacement for chronic mitral regurgitation. Circulation 1991; 84 (Suppl II):II 578.

57. Wong CYH, Spotnitz HM. Systolic and diastolic properties of the human left ventricle during valve replacement for chronic mitral regurgitation. Am J Cardiol 1981; 47:40-50.

58. Urschel CW, Covell JW, Sonnenblick EH et al. Myocardial mechanics in aortic and mitral valvular regurgitation. The concept of instantaneous impedance as a determinant of the performance of the intact heart. J Clin Invest 1968; 47:867-83.

59. Braunwald E. Mitral regurgitation physiological, clinical, surgical considerations. N Engl J Med 1969; 281:425-33.

60. Cohn KE, Rao BS, Russel JA. Force generation and shortening capabilities of left ventricular myocardium in primary and secondary forms of mitral regurgitation. Br Heart J 1969; 31:474-9.

61. Goldfine HL, Aurigemma GP, Gaasch WH. Mechanism of reduction in ejection fraction following mitral valve replacement for mitral regurgitation. Circulation 1992; 86 (Suppl I):I 660.

62. Spratt JA, Olsen CO, Tyson GS et al. Experimental mitral regurgitation: Physiological effects of correction on left ventricular dynamics. J Thorac Cardiovasc Surg 1983; 86:479-89.

63. Harpole Jr DH, Rankin S, Wolfe WG et al. Effects of standard mitral valve replacement on left ventricular function. Ann Thorac Surg 1990; 49:866-74.

64. Gaasch WH, Zile MR. Left ventricular function after surgical correction of chronic mitral regurgitation. Eur Heart J 1991; 12 (Suppl B):48-51.

65. Boucher CA, Bingham JB, Osbakken MD et al. Early changes in left ventricular size and function after correction of ventricular volume overload. Am J Cardiol 1981; 47:991-1004.

66. Kazama S, Nishiguchi K, Sonoda K et al. Postoperative left ventricular function in patients with mitral stenosis. The effect of commissurotomy and valve replacement on left ventricular systolic function. Jpn Heart J 1986; 27:35-42.

67. Sarris GE, Miller DC. Role of the mitral subvalvular apparatus in left ventricular systolic mechanics. Semin Thorac Cardiovasc Surg 1989; 1:133-43.

CHAPTER 4

MITRAL VALVE REPAIR

THE FLOPPY MITRAL VALVE SYNDROME

Since clinical aspects of mitral disease are not the topic of this merely surgical monograph, only a few words will be addressed to the so-called billowing or floppy mitral valve syndrome.[1]

The identification of a billowing or prolapsing mitral valve in patients presenting with nonpathognomonic symptoms is crucial to decide whether medical or surgical therapy is indicated. Most patients present with palpitations and/or atypical chest pain associated with anxiety. In some patients there is no apparent cause of anxiety Often coronary artery disease is suspected. Electrocardiographic stress tests permit a differential diagnosis. It is known that post-exercise ST segment and T wave changes in floppy mitral are almost always different from those due to myocardial ischemia.[2] Moreover since some symptoms—palpitations, chest pain, dyspnea, reduced exercise tolerance, asthenia, syncope, orthostatic hypotension, anxiety—cannot be explained by valve alterations alone, neuroendocrine dysfunction has been suggested.

In a recent review of various aspects of mitral valve prolapse, Boudoulas[3] reported neuroendocrine alterations associated with this syndrome. The author found abnormally high excretion of epinephrine and norepinephrine in symptomatic patients with mitral valve prolapse, and the frequency of ventricular extrasystoles positively correlated with catecholamine excretion.

Abnormal onset of dose related symptoms, such as chest pain, dyspnea, panic attacks, was associated with isoproterenol infusion.[4] An interesting hypothesis was proposed to explain chest pain. The increased heart rate produced by adrenergic stimulation, such as isoproterenol infusion, or spontaneously in cases of supraventricular tachycardia, causes marked reduction of diastolic time that is significantly greater in mitral valve prolapse than in control population. And since subendocardial coronary blood flow is predominantly diastolic, a significant reduction of diastolic time can result in myocardial ischemia producing chest pain.[4]

A central anatomic nervous system defect was suggested by Coghlan[5] and Gaffney.[6] They observed abnormal responses to various stimulations such as Valsalva maneuver, phenylephrine infusion, lower body negative pressure, orthostatic stress, and dive test. They also found that reduced plasma volume in symptomatic patients that can account for the orthostatic tachycardia and hypotension observed in these patients.

These observations suggest a complex pathogenesis of floppy mitral valve syndrome. Indeed abnormalities were observed in responsive to catecholamine levels, vagal tone, baroreceptor control and plasma volume regulation.

Often when only a billowing of the leaflets is present the patient requires reassurance only,[3,7] although a possible underlying pathology, such as Marfan's syndrome or hypertrophic cardiomyopathy, should be excluded.

Ventricular arrhythmias associated with floppy valves can be serious. When these patients have redundant and myxomatous leaflets, real prolapse is often present and risk of severe arrhythmias increases as does that of other complications such as systemic emboli, endocarditis, progressive valve regurgitation, and heart failure.[3,7]

Arrhythmias may vary from atrial ectopic beats to ventricular tachycardia and even ventricular fibrillation with sudden death. The most common rhythm disturbance is ventricular extrasystoles. Patients with this disorder should undergo medical treatment with the most appropriate anti-arrhythmic drug.

Antithrombotic therapy is indicated in cases of systemic embolization. This complication is rare and usually mild since emboli originate from small deposits of fibrin and platelets on the surface of redundant myxomatous leaflets. However coronary artery embolization may explain the cases of myocardial infarction with normal coronary arteries in presence of a floppy mitral valve.[1]

Prophylaxis for infective endocarditis is indicated in advanced cases of billowing leaflets and in any case of mitral regurgitation.

The progression of pathological alterations from minor billowing to significant regurgitation, although described, is not inevitable. Various studies report a wide range of results since the start- and end-points were different and also since the length of the follow-up varied. The incidence of progression to severe mitral regurgitation varied from 5%[8] to more than 15%[9]; this discrepancy may reflect different indications for and timing of surgery.

TIMING OF SURGERY

The best time for a patient with mitral valve disease to undergo surgery is still moot,

regardless of the type of treatment indicated. Many factors contribute to this controversy, from the various etiologies to the different lesions produced, from the various parameters analyzed to predict the results of treatment to the lack of homogeneous groups of patients utilized to compare different medical and surgical treatments.

Peterson[10] reviewed recent studies to identify the best timing for mitral surgery. Functional class is still a factor in mitral stenosis. Yet with conservative procedures such as "closed technique", open-heart commissurotomy or balloon commissurotomy, patients with significant valve stenosis, although in New York Heart Association (NYHA) functional class II, should now be referred for surgery since operative risk is very low. Conversely when echocardiographic findings of heavy leaflet calcification or subvalvular apparatus alterations indicate the need for valve replacement, patients should undergo surgery when they are NYHA functional class III, especially if they are young.[7]

A different approach should be utilized in cases of chronic mitral regurgitation. Functional class indeed is not always correlated with severity of the lesion and ventricular impairment. Other parameters are predictive of postoperative results, such as ejection fraction, end-systolic volume, mean pulmonary pressure or, as recently reported by Wisenbaugh and co-workers,[11] end-systolic diameter. The author observed that survival and symptomatic improvement could be expected if surgical procedure is performed before the left ventricle reaches 50 mm of end-systolic diameter. Also in this type of lesion, when a valve repair is indicated, patients should undergo surgery well before the onset of significant ventricular damage.

In mixed lesions, stenosis plus insufficiency, the likelihood of satisfactory long-lasting valve repair is low. For this reason patients with this type of lesion should undergo surgery only when in NYHA functional class III. Similar conclusions were drawn by Antunes.[12] Analyzing his recent experience, the author observed that more than 80% of mitral operations resulted in valve repair. This was the result in 90% of patients with rheumatic regurgitation, in almost all degenerative cases and in 75-80% of those with rheumatic stenosis. For this reason Antunes suggested early referral for surgery, before NYHA functional class III is reached. Patients with mixed lesions should have surgery before symptomatic deterioration, since the probability of satisfactory valve repair is low in his experience.

Frater[13] compared 60 consecutive patients in whom he reached a decision for valve repair or replacement after 20 minutes devoted to repair with another 60 consecutive patients in whom repair was undertaken regardless of the difficulties encountered and the time required. In the latter group the valve was replaced only when repair failed. The second approach led to more repaired valves without increased operative risk. But when repair failed, aortic crossclamping time necessarily was increased—which could be safely maintained only with excellent cardioplegia and careful removal of air from the ventricle and ascending aorta.

Barlow[7] reported on surgical therapy in cases of life-threatening arrhythmias associated with mild mitral regurgitation. He recommends early referral for surgery even in cases of "nonsurgical" valve incompetence if associated with major ventricular arrhythmias or if there is a history of syncope. Shah,[14] on the other hand, considers this approach drastic and suggests treatment with antiarrhythmic agents.

As has been observed in all First World Countries, in the last eight years we have seen a significant decrease in rheumatic valve disease. Yet expanded application of echocardiography to follow asymptomatic patients with incidentally-discovered mitral prolapse produced a significant increase in the number of patients referred for surgery before the onset of significant symptoms. In our experience this, as well as the increasing confidence in reparative techniques and the development of new procedures, such as artificial chordae insertion, has led to a significant increase in mitral valve repair versus replacement—from about 30% in the early 80s to about 80% in the early 90s. Considering only cases of degenerative pathology, more than 90% are repaired now.

EXPERIMENTAL AND CLINICAL EXPERIENCES

Since the early 50s "closed" treatment of mitral stenosis has achieved satisfactory results. On the other hand, many attempts to correct mitral regurgitation have been undertaken, before a reliable valve prosthesis was clinically available,[15] with inconstant results and significant risk.[16]

In accordance with the suggestions of Wilson and Murray and co-workers in 1938,[17-18] in the early 50s—before cardiopulmonary by-pass was available—many surgeons tried to reduce the hemodynamic effects of mitral regurgitation by focusing on the valve annulus, leaflets and orifice. They suggested decreasing annulus size or approximating the commissures.[19-23] Leaflet tissue was replaced with biological or artificial materials[17,19,22,24-26] or the regurgitant orifice was obliterated the with slings (autologous tendon, fascia lata, vein, pericardium) pushed through the valve by systolic pressure,[27-29] or with artificial sponges placed across the valve.[30-32] Since most of these procedures were performed externally approach without cardiopulmonary by-pass, pathology of the subvalvular apparatus was not considered correctable.

After the introduction of extracorporeal circulation some of the previous techniques were modified for the open approach,[33-36] while new procedures were tested to improve results. Attention focused on correction of mitral regurgitation due to chordal rupture.

In October 1958 McGoon performed the first plication of the posterior leaflet for chordal rupture without resection and without annuloplasty,[37,38] followed by a large series of similar procedures—mainly plication of one or both commissures—in most of which annuloplasty was performed.[36]

Another field of research grew out of Wilson's experimental paper of 1930[18] regarding the implantation of autologous pericardium inside the heart. Afterward Bakst and co-workers,[26] Sauvage and co-workers,[39,40] and Frater and co-workers[41-43] produced clinical experiences with extension or replacement of leaflet and chordal tissue by fresh autologous pericardium. Clinical results were often less encouraging when compared with experimental reports, until tanning procedures of pericardial sheets became available.[44]

The first successful clinical experience with a valve prosthesis was reported by Starr and Edwards in 1961,[15] and most researchers and surgeons directed their attention to find the best valve substitute. Other surgeons focused their efforts to improve surgical techniques and methods of myocardial protection for mitral valve replacement. The greatest influence on mitral valve reconstruction was contributed by Carpentier, who standardized most of the surgical techniques still utilized in mitral repair.[45-52] His description of ring annuloplasty in 1968[45] and the "functional approach" described in 1978[47] represented two majors steps in rationalizing and standardizing this procedure.

Carpentier's Honored Guest's Address, read at the Annual Meeting of the American Association for Thoracic Surgery, in Atlanta in 1983, entitled "Cardiac Valve Surgery— the "French Correction,"[49] was a brilliant account of valve repair. In this lecture he summarized the state-of-the-art of this procedure based on his wide experience. First, with the "functional approach" he significantly simplified the classification of mitral valve pathology, distinguishing only two functional alterations: increased and restricted leaflet motion. The recognition of the type of functional alteration of each leaflet was essential to successful surgery.

Systematic sequential examination of the valve apparatus was described, starting with annular size. The leaflet tissue is then analyzed for qualitative and dynamic changes. Since the posterior leaflet segment close to the anterolateral commissure is often nonprolapsing, this area is utilized as a "reference point"[49,53] to evaluate the relative motion of the different components of leaflet tissue. In cases of mitral regurgitation coexisting with normal leaflet excursion, primary annular dilatation or leaflet perforation should be noted. Once increased leaflet motion, i.e., prolapse, is identified, chordal or papillary muscle elongation or rupture should be sought, while restricted leaflet motion may indicate commissural tissue fusion or thickening of any of the valve components, leaflets or chordae.

Several operative procedures were suggested by Carpentier. For posterior leaflet prolapse, rectangular resection is the procedure of choice to prevent chordal elongation or rupture, or leaflet perforation. The leaflet is reconstructed by plication of the annulus and approximation of the leaflet stumps. yet reconstruction of rectangular leaflet resection can be associated with systolic anterior motion of the mitral valve, producing left ventricular outflow tract obstruction, during the early postoperative period in some cases of prosthetic ring annuloplasty.[54,55] Redundant posterior leaflet tissue or an oversized prosthetic ring are predisposing factors. Consequently a modification of the rectangular resection was proposed to reduce the height of the redundant posterior leaflet and to obviate the need for excessive annular plication to repair large tissue resections: the "sliding leaflet technique."[50,55,56] After resecting the area of pathologic chordal support, the residual posterior leaflet is partially detached from the annulus and sutured in such a way that the "sliding tissue" is reduced in height and is pushed in order to obliterate the defect produced by resection, simultaneously avoiding large annular plications (Fig. 4.1).

Regarding the anterior leaflet, triangular resection of pathological areas was attempted in early repair experience.[36,49,50,57] The results were not encouraging and this procedure was abandoned.[49,50] Prolapse of the anterior leaflet is generally caused by chordal lesions, and several techniques were suggested to correct these alterations.[49] When chordal rupture is present, two options were suggested by Carpentier: fixation of the unsupported free edge to adjacent strong secondary chordae (Fig. 4.2), if present, or anterior transposition of normal chordae of the posterior leaflet facing the pathological area of the anterior leaflet (Fig. 4.3).

In cases of chordal elongation, shortening is performed by invagination into a pouch created by splitting the corresponding papillary muscle. When mitral regurgitation is present as a result of chordal elongation or, as in some cases of leaflet perforation is due to leaflet tissue insufficiency secondary to

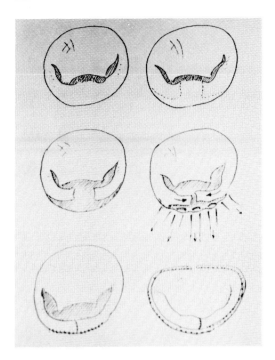

Fig. 4.1. The "sliding leaflet technique" utilized to reduce the height of a redundant posterior leaflet, avoiding possible anterior displacement of the anterior leaflet, with consequent left ventricular outflow obstruction, in case of rigid ring application for mitral annuloplasty. The same technique obviates the need for large annular plication in case of extensive quadrangular resection. (From A.Carpentier The SAM issue. Le Club Mitrale Newsletter 1989; 1:5. Reproduced with permission from the author and Promedica International Publisher).

endocarditis, Carpentier utilized glutaraldehyde tanned autologous pericardium to replace the tissue defect.[51,52]

As mentioned, in 1968 Carpentier introduced the prosthetic ring annuloplasty, thought to be essential in most cases of mitral regurgitation.[45-46,49,50] The rigid device conceived by the author has two major features: it reestablishes the correct valve orifice area and reshapes the annular conformation. Indeed, in chronic mitral regurgitation, significant orifice enlargement is associated with "circularization" of the valve surface that alters the ratio between anteroposterior and transverse diameters that is normally 3:4.[50] With Carpentier's prosthetic ring implantation the normal conformation is restored. We already discussed the problem of anterior

displacement of the valve, producing left ventricular outflow tract obstruction, in some cases of prosthetic ring annuloplasty, and the consequent solution suggested by Carpentier,[50-55] and we will extend the discussion in the chapter dedicated to the different options available for mitral annuloplasty, associated with artificial chordae implantation.

Other surgeons devoted their research and clinical experience to improve the techniques and expand the indications for mitral reconstruction. Frater and co-workers, after carefully analyzing the functional anatomy of the mitral apparatus, tested and clinically utilized different materials to replace portions of the mitral apparatus—leaflet and/or chordae—during valve repair.[41-43,58-60] To perform these procedures they established a few fundamental anatomical rules (Fig. 4.4).

(1) Cusp tissue is never interrupted all around the annulus, and its area must be larger than the mitral orifice at the end of systole.

(2) The free margins of the main anterior and posterior cusps are suspended at the same level relative to each other in the ventricular cavity, throughout cardiac cycle, and the sum of the heights of the two leaflets must exceed the diameter of the relaxed ring.

(3) Chordae tendineae should be under tension both in diastole and systole to maintain the leaflets in proper position. Their length should be less than the distance from their papillary attachment to the valve annular plane, preventing the free edges of the leaflets from reaching this plane in systole.

All these suggestions were used by the authors in a series of animal experiments and clinical applications reported in 1965.[43] They utilized untreated autologous pericardium to extend or replace atrioventricular valve leaflets and chordae.

Experimental specimens showed fibrin deposition and cellular infiltration, mostly by macrophages, starting in the early postoperative period, while, with time, pericardium thickened and shrunk and, after two months, lost pliability, with extensive tissue hyalinization. Also cartilage formation could be detected, increasing in frequency over time.

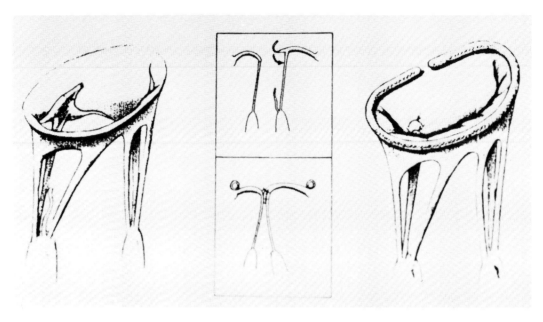

Fig. 4.2. Fixation of the unsupported free edge of the anterior leaflet to adjacent strong secondary chordae, if present, in cases of chordal rupture. (From A. Carpentier. Cardiac valve surgery—the "French correction." J Thorac Cardiovasc Surg 1983; 86:323-37. Reproduced with the permission from the author and Mosby-Year Book, Inc.).

The clinical series provided better short term results, since the specimens retrieved up to two months after implantation showed minimal change, but a mitral patch removed after 15 months for recurrent mitral regurgitation had extensive myxomatous degeneration. Also most patients, although with a satisfactory repair exemplified by disappearance of any murmur and improvement of functional class, had early recurrence of regurgitation when a mitral extension patch was used.[43]

For these reasons, for many years Frater and co-workers tested various materials to replace leaflet and/or chordae of the mitral valve (Fig 4.5 and 4.6), in order to find the best substitute capable of creating a competent valve, to maintain valve dimensions, and to heal to papillary muscle and leaflet tissue while still retaining flexibility.[59] They utilized autologous, homologous, and xenograft pericardium fresh, or treated by glutaraldehyde or glycerol, both in animal models (dog and sheep) and clinical use.[41,59,61-65] Also the influence of the site of implantation—atrial wall, leaflet, chordae, aortic wall, pericardium—

was evaluated with regard to stress and thrombogenicity.[62,64]

In animal models, glutaraldehyde-treated xenograft pericardium (bovine) used as a chordae substitute maintained the length, but showed considerable stiffening that did not significantly impair leaflet motion as long as only one chorda had been replaced leaving residual normal chordae in place. Histological examination revealed changes not significantly different from those found in fresh autologous pericardium: by four months fibrosis was detected, while calcification, cartilage, and bone formation were present after one year.[59] Comparing untreated versus briefly treated autologous pericardium in chordal positions in dogs, the authors[63] found that both materials maintained length. Pliability was present in the middle portion of treated chordae, while untreated specimens were stiff and less pliable throughout. Healing was satisfactory at both ends in the two groups. Histologically the changes were of the same type but with different distribution: a thick fibrous sheath uniformly covered fresh chordae, while it was confined to the ends in

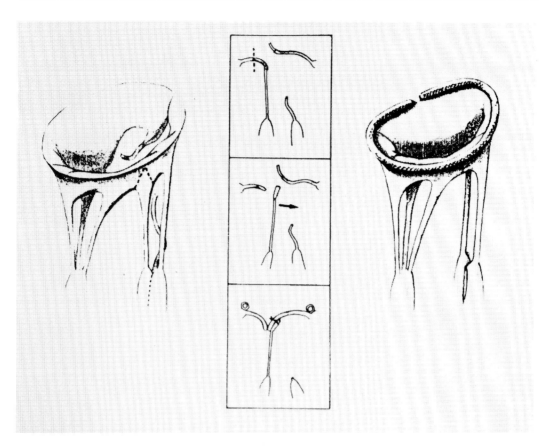

Fig. 4.3. Transposition of normal posterior chordae to support the anterior leaflet in case of anterior chordal rupture. (From A. Carpentier. Cardiac valve surgery—the "French correction." J Thorac Cardiovasc Surg 1983; 86:323-37. Reproduced with permission from the author and Mosby-Year Book, Inc.).

Fig 4.4. Rules proposed by Frater to achieve satisfactory mitral valve repair. Normal mitral valve (frames A and B) and mechanisms of valve regurgitation (frames C and D). A=length of anterior cusp of mitral valve; B=distance from the distal attachment of chordae tendineae to the valve ring; C=distance from the distal attachment of chordae tendineae to the free edge of the leaflet; D=diameter of mitral valve ring; P=length of posterior cusp of the mitral valve; X-Y=plane of the level to which the main cusps descend. (From RWM Frater et al. Reproducible replacement of elongated or ruptured mitral valve chordae. Ann Thorac Surg 1983; 35:14-28. Reproduced with permission of the author, of the Society of Thoracic Surgeons and Elsevier Science Publishing Co, Inc.).

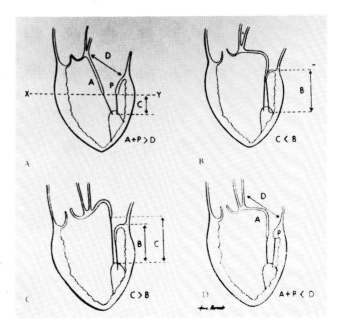

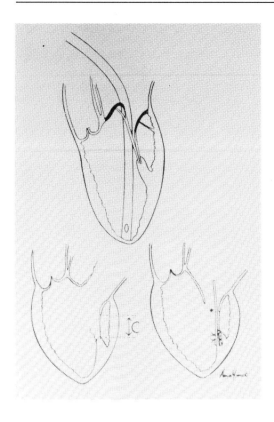

Fig. 4.5. Stages in the replacement of a main anterior cusp chorda. A suction catheter is used to fix the apex of the arrested heart to determine true prolapse (top). With this procedure, the free edge of the anterior cusp is at the same level in the ventricle as the free edge of the posterior cusp (bottom). C=distance from the point of distal attachment of chordae tendineae to the free edge of the valve. (From RWM Frater et al. Reproducible replacement of elongated or ruptured mitral valve chordae. Ann Thorac Surg 1983; 35:14-28. Reproduced with permission of the author, of the Society of Thoracic Surgeons and Elsevier Science Publishing Co, Inc.).

treated chordae. Calcifications and cartilage formation were present at both ends in treated specimens, mostly on the papillary muscle side in untreated chordae, while collagen degeneration was uniform and severe in treated cases and less severe in untreated specimens. In two cases, one from each group, the artificial chorda disconnected from the leaflet attachment and in both cases pericardium was completely retracted loosing its original length and shape.

The last observation suggested the role of tension in maintaining the length and preventing progressive alterations of pericardial chordae, regardless of treatment. The protective effect of stress forces was confirmed in another series of experiments[62] in which the same material, glutaraldehyde-tanned bovine pericardium, was implanted in various positions in a canine model. Indeed, while in the chordal position its length was preserved and it became stiff and calcified only at the ends, maintaining pliability in the central area, when utilized as an atrial wall patch, without pressure or tension stress, the pericardium shrunken and calcified extensively, with bone formation in most cases.

In a complete review of their experience, the authors described the role of various materials, fixation methods, and sites of implantation.[64] When suspended into the right atrium without significant stress, short-term glutaraldehyde-fixed autologous pericardium was satisfactorily preserved without significant distinction from long-term tanned xenograft pericardium, while short-term fixed homologous pericardium degenerated markedly. This suggests an immune response to incompletely tanned homologous tissue. In chordal positions, under continuous tensile stress, no significant differences could be found in terms of healing and preservation of length between tanned autologous and xenograft pericardium, although the fibrous covering, which stiffened all specimens, seemed more pronounced in xenograft specimens.

A "cuspal effect" was suggested by the severe degeneration and early calcification of xenograft pericardium used for leaflet extension where stress conditions should be quite

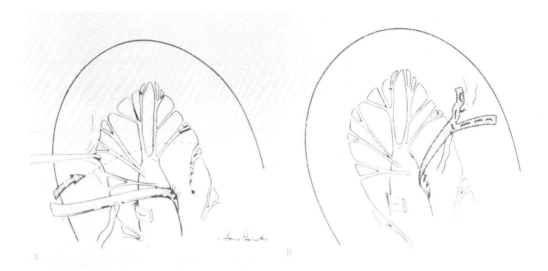

Fig. 4.6. Chordal replacement with a pericardial strip. Anterolateral side of the mitral valve with ruptured main chordae of left side of anterior cusp. (A) A pericardial strip has been stitched to the papillary muscle and a marker stitch has been placed in the pericardium to indicate the level of the posterior cusp opposite the point where the anterior cusp meets it. (B) The strip is attached to the anterior cusp. The marker stitch is at the level of the free edge of the anterior cusp. (From RWM Frater et al. Reproducible replacement of elongated or ruptured mitral valve chordae. Ann Thorac Surg 1983; 35:14-28. Reproduced with permission of the author, of the Society of Thoracic Surgeons and Elsevier Science Publishing Co, Inc.).

similar to those in chordal positions. Moreover, an "atrial factor" was postulated as responsible for the marked fibrotic and calcific changes observed when xenograft pericardium was used as an atrial wall patch, in conditions of very low pressure and tensile stress. In the aortic wall position both tanned autologous and xenograft pericardium behaved satisfactorily, with minimal alterations and without any aneurysmal dilatation.

In conclusion, site of utilization and immune reactions seem to play a significant role in the behavior of tanned pericardium. A stress load seems to better preserve structure and function. Autologous, homologous, and xenograft pericardium behave similarly when they are glutaraldehyde tanned for an adequate period of time. Varying results may reflect different sites or conditions of implantation.[66]

The same laboratory, attempted mitral valve repair utilizing material treated with sterile 98% glycerol.[65] This is a poor tanning agent, and it does not prevent an immune reaction by the host. Moreover it cannot be considered a sterilizing agent since many sporigenous bacteria can survive its application. It partially dehydrates the pericardium, making it stiff, but it recovers its normal pliability with saline rinsing, so glycerol-treated pericardium may be considered a "living tissue."[65] In chordal or leaflet patch positions, it healed fairly well and retained its original dimensions and flexibility.

Histologically the graft was covered by a fibrous sheath infiltrated with mononuclear cells. Focal calcification and cartilage formation was observed in the cuspal position. Pericardium showed progressive fragmentation and reabsorption of collagen fibers, until only the overgrown fibrous tissue remained without any residual pericardial elements. This interesting observation suggested that glycerol-treated pericardium might used as a mold for autologous tissue growth to replace pathological structures.

Many other experiences were reported with fresh autologous tissues such as pericardium[67-69] or fascia lata[70-72] without encouraging results, similar to those reported by Frater's group.

The successful introduction of glutaraldehyde tanning of bioprostheses by

Carpentier[44] resulted in the application of glutaraldehyde-tanned bovine pericardium in mitral valve reconstruction. But long-term results were poor due to graft calcification.

In the attempt to avoid simultaneously immune and degenerative alterations observed with fresh materials, since 1980 Carpentier's group has utilized glutaraldehyde-tanned autologous pericardium for leaflet extension, mostly in rheumatic cases.[52] The results have been; no graft calcifications could be detected in cases requiring reoperation up to six years after implantation, although 12% of the patients required reoperation, mostly for progression of disease.

In children graft failure is absent although it occurs routinely, with early calcification, with other bioprostheses. Other authors could not confirm this striking difference between the behavior of treated autologous and xenograft pericardium.[66,73]

A review of their experience in techniques of leaflet advancement was recently reported by Hisatomi et al.[74] Utilizing fresh autologous or glutaraldehyde-tanned xenograft pericardium to extend mitral leaflets in patients mostly affected by rheumatic valve pathology (69% of the cases), they observed reoperation rates of 10.5% at five years, and 36.2% at ten years. Distinguishing patients with preoperative pure mitral regurgitation from those with mitral stenosis alone or associated with regurgitation, signs of valve dysfunction were absent in 90% of cases at five years and in 69.1% at ten years in the former group, but only in 62.5% at five years, and 25% at ten years in the latter group. Patch calcifications could be detected in 3 of the 13 patients that required reoperation, more than nine years after the original procedure with no difference between autologous and xenograft pericardium. The authors concluded that leaflet advancement is a satisfactory procedure for mitral regurgitation, although valve dysfunction recurs early when mitral stenosis is present.

A considerable contribution to the mitral valve repair experience was also provided by Duran's group.[75,76] Besides amplifying the techniques for chordal shortening, they pro-

posed the utilization of a different device for prosthetic ring annuloplasty, a flexible ring. The characteristics of this device will be discussed in the chapter dedicated to annular procedures.

In a recent paper Duran reviewed all techniques currently utilized to repair chordae elongation.[77] Chordal shortening by papillary muscle sliding was originally described by Carpentier and consists of vertically splitting the papillary muscle for a length corresponding to the amount of chordal elongation. The tip of the papillary muscle connected to elongated chordae is then sutured to a lower level of the other half of the papillary muscle. With thin, difficult to split papillary muscles or with elongated chordae arising from different muscle heads, the "looping" technique can be utilized (Fig. 4.7). A loop around the base of the elongated chorda is formed with a double-armed suture. Then the two strands of the suture are passed through the papillary muscle and secured down toward the base of the muscle to obtain a loop of the elongated chorda lying against the side of the muscle.

When elongated chordae arise as a group from a single papillary muscle head, this structure can be lowered suturing the head to a lower level of a contiguous papillary muscle (Fig. 4.8).

With the "flip-over" transposition a square of the normal posterior leaflet opposite to the pathological anterior chordae is identified, resected, and mobilized by dividing second order chordae. This tissue is then superimposed over the anterior leaflet, with the ventricular surface toward the atrium so that the free edge of the transposed segment can be sutured to the free edge of the anterior leaflet and the annular portion to the atrial surface of the same leaflet (Fig. 4.9). The posterior resection is then closed as a usual rectangular resection.

Another technique suggested by Duran in cases of diffuse chordal elongation is plication at the leaflet side. The elongated chorda is bent and the resulting loop is fastened to the atrial surface of the free edge of the leaflet.

Comparing their experience in treating

mitral insufficiency with valve repair versus replacement with bioprosthesis, Duran and co-workers had a significantly lower operative mortality in the repair group (1.9% versus 11.4%). Since this was a retrospective, nonrandomized study,[75] this difference could be related to the surgical indications. The results suggest early operation (functional class II) when repair was indicated and delay when a replacement was more likely necessary. Nevertheless when the results were evaluated by preoperative functional class, a significant difference was observed in operative mortality between class III and IV patients who underwent valve repair versus those undergoing valve replacement. A significant difference in late results (mortality,

thromboembolism, valve dysfunction) could not be discerned.

Similar results were reported by Yacoub and co-workers,[57] comparing valve repair with valve replacement (inverted, fresh, unstented, antibiotic sterilized aortic homograft). Early mortality was lower after repair (3.1% versus 7%) and also late survival was significantly better in this group of patients (90% versus 62% at five years). In this series satisfactory long-term hemodynamic results after valve repair were reported although a prosthetic ring was never used. A systolic murmur was present in half of the cases early after operation and it persisted during the follow-up.

Orszulak and co-workers reviewed Mayo

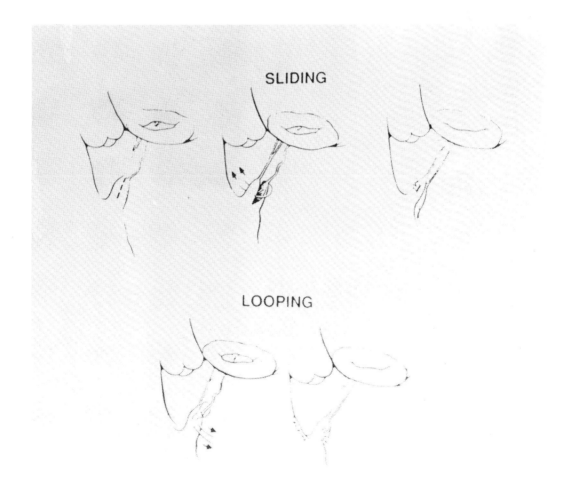

Fig. 4.7. Comparison between "sliding" and "looping" techniques to shorten elongated chordae, mostly in cases of thin papillary muscles. (From CG Duran. Surgical management of elongated chordae of the mitral valve. J Cardiac Surg 1989; 4:253-9. Reproduced with permission of the author and Futura Publishing Co, Inc.).

Clinic experience in the treatment of mitral regurgitation due to ruptured chordae tendineae.[36] Comparing repair versus replacement they could not find a significant difference in early mortality, while late survival was significantly better in the repair group. The incidence of thromboembolism was lower in this group (1.8% vs 8.0% patient-years). In this series the probability of reoperation increased with time after repair, contrary to other experiences in which reoperations were performed early after repair.[57] This late manifestation of recurrent regurgitation indicates progression of the pathology mitigating the beneficial effect of annuloplasty (commissural plication in more than 95% of the cases) and leading to leaflet prolapse and chordal rupture. Based on this experience the authors suggested the need for utilization of more reliable annuloplasty techniques. This is beneficial as well in cases of leaflet resection associated with minimal or absent annular dilatation since reduction of the valve orifice decreases tensile stress on the repaired leaflet, avoiding suture dehiscence.[36]

The importance of annuloplasty was emphasized also by Cosgrove.[78] This procedure is considered an integral part of most mitral valve repair since it produces many effects: it corrects annular dilatation, when present; prevents further dilatation; decreases the likelihood of dehiscence of the sutures utilized to fix leaflet resection; and optimizes coaptation of the leaflets. Reviewing 650 mitral repairs for pure valve regurgitation, the author reported an incidence of valvuloplasty of 75% in cases of degenerative etiology, of 68% for ischemic disease, and about 50% when congenital, rheumatic or infective disease was the cause of mitral insufficiency.[78] Moreover he demonstrated a learning curve that accounts for the fact that in about 20% of cases in 1980 valves were repaired whereas in 1988 repair accounted for about 70% of all mitral procedures. In fact, 88% of degenerated valves were repaired in 1988. The results also confirmed a lower early operative mortality for valvuloplasty when compared with valve replacement (4% versus 8%) for any etiology. Also in this regard, data were particularly significant for degenerative disease: 2.4% versus 10% operative mortality for valve repair and replacement, respectively.

These results go a long way to overcome the concern of increased risk of longer aortic crossclamping time required when a valve is repaired rather than replaced. With current methods of myocardial protection, this drawback is greatly mitigated by preservation of ventricular function that contributes to improved long-term survival, a better functional

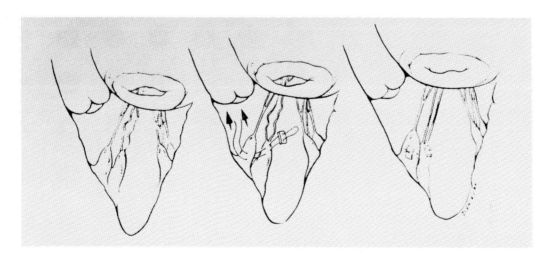

Fig. 4.8. Papillary head repositioning in case of many elongated chordae arising from the same papillary muscle head. (From CG Duran. Surgical management of elongated chordae of the mitral valve. J Cardiac Surg 1989; 4:253-9. Reproduced with permission of the author and Futura Publishing Co, Inc.).

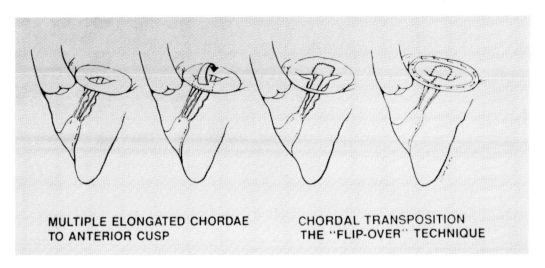

**MULTIPLE ELONGATED CHORDAE
TO ANTERIOR CUSP**

**CHORDAL TRANSPOSITION
THE "FLIP-OVER" TECHNIQUE**

Fig. 4.9. The "flip-over" technique is a modification of the chordal transposition technique illustrated in Figure 3. A square of mitral posterior leaflet is transposed, reversed, over the facing pathological anterior leaflet. (From CG Duran. Surgical management of elongated chordae of the mitral valve. J Cardiac Surg 1989; 4:253-9. Reproduced with permission of the author and Futura Publishing Co, Inc.).

result, a lower incidence of endocarditis, and a lower rate of thromboembolism.[78]

An important contribution to the literature regarding long-term results after mitral valvuloplasty is anticipated from Carpentier's group.

Deloche and co-workers[50] reported the experience of a 15-year follow-up with most of the currently used techniques. The authors focused particularly on two major issues still controversial due to the extreme heterogeneity of patient population, timing of surgery, technique utilized, and follow-up methods: (1) predictability of the technique and (2) consistency of the results. Regarding the first point, they reported a 4% incidence of early reoperation, mostly due to residual prolapse, extensive anterior leaflet triangular resection, or omission of ring annuloplasty. With improvements in indications and techniques, most of these reoperations should be avoided today. Indeed extensive use of transesophageal echocardiography to evaluate the areas of prolapse, utilization of posterior chordae transposition and regular performance of ring annulolasty, associated with the "sliding posterior leaflet technique", produced a significant reduction in these complications and the subsequent need for early reoperation. Consistency of the results is supported by a

92.7% reoperation-free rate for patients with degenerative valve disease, and 76.1% reoperation-free ratefor those with rheumatic disease. Interestingly, at 15-year follow-up the survival rate was better in patients with rheumatic disease (81.1% versus 71.2%), probably because they were young and their left ventricles were not so severely compromised, while no differences could be detected if valve-related deaths were considered alone. In any acse, the authors estimated the lieklihood of successful repair to be about 95%, 75%, and 70% for degenerative, ischemic, and rheumatic mitral valve disease, respectively.

In two recent papers, the same group of authors[51,79] reported experience with mitral valve repair in two particular situations. In the first report[51] they analyzed the outcome of early operation in cases of acute endocarditis. They utilized all Carpentier's techniques, including glutaraldehyde-fixed autologous pericardium patch application to repair leaflet tissue lacking due to infective perforation or surgical excision, but avoiding prosthetic ring annuloplasty any time it was feasible.

The results confirmed the safety and efficacy of early surgery. Indeed only one early death (2.5%) and one late death were reported, with one early reoperation for dehiscence of posterior quadrangular resection and no instances of recurrent endocarditis, regardless of the type of etiologic agent or preoperative antibiotic regimen. Early repair reduces tissue damage and the need for biological or artificial prosthetic materials, and preserves left ventricular function.

In the second paper the authors[79] analyzed their experience with mitral valvuloplasty, mostly for degenerative disease, in elderly patients (more than 70 years). Operative mortality of 3.8%, with a five-year survival of 81 ±11%, associated with freedom from thromboembolism, hemorrhage, and reoperation of 97%, 97%, and 98%, respectively, demonstrated that advanced age is not a contradiction of valve repair. It is best option to preserve ventricular function in order to improve early and late results.

SURGERY FOR CHORDAL ALTERATIONS

In addition to the techniques reported by Carpentier (Fig. 4.2 and 4.3), Frater (Fig. 4.5 and 4.6) and Duran (Fig. 4.7-4.9), a series of recent papers reviewed different techniques and clinical experiences, particularly regarding the treatment of chordal elongation or rupture.[53,77,80-85] A paper from the Mayo Clinic[36] reported the long-term follow-up with the "leaflet plication technique without excision"[37] and all the other various associatedprocedures. Follow-up data were described here previously.

In 1986 Hvass et al[80] reported their experience with posterior chordae transposition to the anterior leaflet, in cases of extensive anterior chordal elongation or rupture. Dealing with the difficulties often related to the treatment of these particular lesions[86] they utilized the transposition associated with other techniques described by Carpentier.[49] Etiology was rheumatic in all cases and many patients were under 15 years of age (8 out of 13). The results were satisfactory, and only one boy required reoperation for retraction of the posterior leaflet, while the transposition had produced a non-prolapsing anterior leaflet. From their experience the authors stressed the need to avoid extensive resection of the posterior leaflet. In any case no more than 25% of this cusp should be dissected.

A major contribution regarding the results obtained with this technique was provided by Lessana and co-workers.[81-87] Since the description by Carpentier in 1983[49] that suggested this method to prevent the poor results obtained with other techniques[47,48,88] the authors utilized partial transposition in cases of ruptured or elongated chordae with rheumatic (55% of the cases), degenerative, infective, or traumatic etiology. They extended the procedure from transposition of a small selected number of chordae to transposition of a portion of the posterior cusp with corresponding chordae. Other maneuvers at annular, leaflet, and chordal levels were utilized as well, when needed. Their observations confirmed the effectiveness of this technique, although etiology significantly influenced short-term results (maximum follow-up 35 months). Actually rheumatic valves accounted for six of the seven patients with significant mitral regurgitation at follow-up (five under 14 years of age) while degenerative and infective lesions had the best outcome.

Discussing this paper, Frater[89] expressed his concern about resecting normal tissue from the posterior leaflet to transpose and move tissue to perform a rectangular resection, often required for the commonly associated mural leaflet pathology. Similar considerations were reported by David.[90] By Doppler echocardiography in these patients, he observed a mean diastolic gradient of 5 mm Hg after chordal transposition probably due to a reduced motion of the repaired segment of the anterior leaflet. In the same discussion, Colvin[91] reported his experience in which he utilized chordal transposition only in cases of chordal rupture near the papillary muscles, while he preferred resuspension to adjacent secondary chordae when rupture was at leaflet level.

A partial modification of the transposition technique was proposed by Cosgrove.[53] Observing that secondary chordae of portions of the posterior leaflet, resected for primary chordae elongation or rupture, are often quite normal, the author suggested utilizing these square segments with secondary chordae in place to transpose to the anterior leaflet or to other close areas of the same posterior leaflet (Fig. 4.10).

Also since chordal alterations progress from mild elongation to rupture, when the long-term integrity of primary attenuated chordae is a concern, Cosgrove's experience suggests replacing them with more normal secondary chordae. These structures are dissected from their leaflet attachment and sutured to the corresponding free edge (Fig. 4.11).

A different approach to correct flail anterior leaflet in mitral or tricuspid position was proposed by Sutlic and co-workers in 1990,[83] with a modification of posterior leaflet and

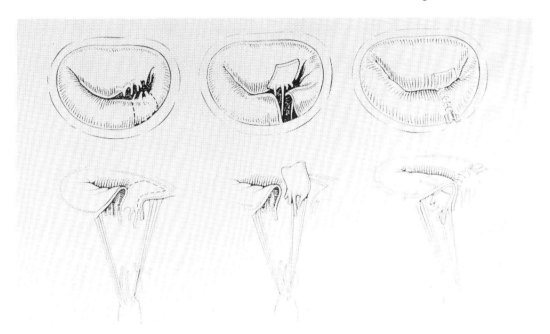

Fig. 4.10. Another modification of the transposition technique utilizes square segments of posterior leaflet, resected for pathology of primary chordae, with normal secondary chordae to be transposed anteriorly. (From DM Cosgrove. Mitral valve repair in patients with elongated chordae tendineae. J Cardiac Surg 1989; 4:247-52. Reproduced with the permission of the author and Futura Publishing Co, Inc.).

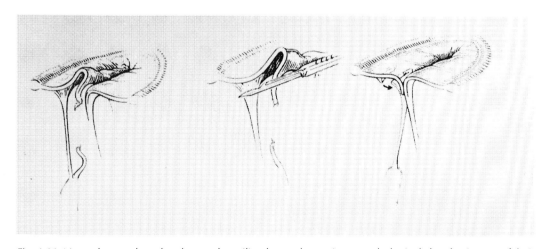

Fig. 4.11. Normal secondary chordae can be utilized to replace primary pathological chordae in case of their rupture or attenuation producing concern about their fate. (From DM Cosgrove. Mitral valve repair in patients with elongated chordae tendineae. J Cardiac Surg 1989; 4:247-52. Reproduced with the permission of the author and Futura Publishing Co, Inc.).

chordae transposition. They excise completely the flail area of the anterior leaflet and detach from the annulus a portion of posterior leaflet for a length corresponding to the height of the stump of anterior leaflet left in place. The mobilized portion of the posterior leaflet is then slid to be sutured to the anterior leaflet, thereby obtaining a different type of transposition. The operation is completed by plicating the portion of annulus deficient of leaflet, without any prosthetic annuloplasty. This technique was proposed for infective chordal rupture since it is advantageous to avoid any prosthetic device in these patients.This was also confirmed in the comment by Jebara et al,[85] although they considered ring implantation mandatory when leaflet resection was wide to reduce tension and prevent suture dehiscence.

Gregory et al[82] proposed an alternative technique for mitral valve repair for ruptured anterior leaflet chordae. They suggested creating a neochorda by dissecting a 5 mm-wide strip of anterior leaflet from the annular insertion to within 5 mm of the free edge, in the area corresponding to the broken chorda. This strip is then reversed into the ventricle and sutured to the papillary muscle while the anterior leaflet is repaired with interrupted sutures. Their experience however was limited to two cases, one requiring valve replacement five years later, for further chordal rupture.

Alvarez et al[92] utilized two other techniques in the event both leaflets were flail in the same area (anterolateral or posteromedial). If the leaflets are not redundant they simply sutured together the free margins of the leaflets. If redundant tissue was present, they superimposed the ventricular surface of the flail posterior leaflet to the anterior leaflet and sutured the anterior free margin to the ventricular surface of the posterior leaflet and the posterior free margin to the atrial surface of the anterior leaflet. To both techniques they added commissural suture annuloplasty. The concern about possible valve stenosis produced by these techniques was overcome by the insignificant gradients observed, although at rest.

All these experiences demonstrate that chordal pathology often conditions the result of valve repair. Also, in some cases, techniques

that utilize only native valve tissue are not adequate to make effective correction and chordal replacement could be the only possible alternative in these instances.

REFERENCES

1. Barlow JB, Pocock WA. Mitral leaflet billowing and prolapse. In: Barlow JB, ed. Perspectives on the mitral valve. Philadelphia: FA Davis Co., 1987:45-112.
2. Barlow JB. The "false-positive" exercise electrocardiogram, value of time course patterns in assessment of depressed ST segments and inverted T waves. Am Heart J 1985; 110:1328-36.
3. Boudoulas H. Mitral valve prolapse: Etiology, clinical presentation and neuroendocrine function. J Heart Valve Dis 1992; 1:175-88.
4. Boudoulas H, Reynolds JC, Mazzaferri E et al. Mitral valve prolapse syndrome: The effect of adrenergic stimulation. J Am Coll Cardiol 1983; 2:638-44.
5. Coghlan CH. Autonomic dysfunction in the mitral valve prolapse syndrome: The brain-heart connection and interaction. In: Boudoulas H, Wooley CF, eds. Mitral valve prolapse and the mitral valve prolapse syndrome. Mount Kisco, NY: Futura Publishing Co., 1988:389-426.
6. Gaffney AF, Blomqvist GC. Mitral valve prolapse and autonomic nervous system dysfunction: A pathophysiological link. In: Boudoulas H, Wooley CF, eds. Mitral valve prolapse and the mitral valve prolapse syndrome. Mount Kisco, NY: Futura Publishing Co., 1988:427-43.
7. Barlow JB. Idiopathic (degenerative) and rheumatic mitral valve prolapse: Historical aspects and an overview. J Heart Valve Dis 1992; 1:163-74.
8. Wilcken DEL, Hickey HA. Lifetime risk of patients with mitral valve prolapse developing severe mitral regurgitation requiring surgery. Circulation 1988; 78:10-4.
9. You-Bing D, Takenaka K, Sakamoto T et al. Follow-up in mitral valve prolapse by phonocardiography, M-mode and two-dimensional echocardiography and Doppler echocardiography. Am J Cardiol 1990; 65:349-54.

10. Peterson KL. Timing of cardiac surgery in chronic mitral valve disease: Implications of natural history studies and left ventricular mechanics. Semin Thorac Cardiovasc Surg 1989; 1:106-17.

11. Wisenbaugh T, Skudicky D, Sareli P. Timing of valve replacement for mitral regurgitation: How soon is too soon and how late is too late? Circulation 1992; 86 (Suppl I):I 497.

12. Antunes MJ. Mitral valve repair into the 1990s. Eur J Cardio-thorac Surg 1992; 6 (Suppl 1):S 13-S 16.

13. Frater RWM. Mitral valvuloplasty. Cardiac Chronicle 1987; 2:1-5.

14. Shah PM. Mitral valve prolapse—The elusive definitions and differing criteria of diagnosis. J Heart Valve Dis 1992; 1:160-2.

15. Starr A, Edwards ML. Mitral replacement: Clinical experience with a ball-valve prosthesis. Ann Surg 1961; 154:726-40.

16. Odell JA, Schurek JO, Barnard CN et al. Long-term results of the Ivalon baffle mitral valve repair. Ann Thorac Surg 1992; 54:283-5.

17. Murray G, Wilkenson FR, Mackenzie R. Reconstruction of the valves of the heart. Can Med Assoc J 1938; 38:317-9.

18. Wilson WC. Studies in experimental mitral obstruction in relation to the surgical treatment of mitral stenosis. Br J Surg 1930; 18:259-74.

19. Bailey CP, Jamison WL, Bakst A et al. The surgical correction of mitral insufficiency by the use of pericardial grafts. J Thorac Surg 1954; 28:551-603.

20. Kay ED, Cross F. The surgical treatment of mitral insufficiency. Surgery 1955; 37:697-706.

21. Sakakibara S. Surgical approach to the correction of mitral insufficiency. Ann Surg 1955; 142:196-203.

22. Nichols HT. Mitral insufficiency: Treatment by polar cross-fusion of the mitral annulus fibrosus. J Thorac Surg 1957; 33:102-22.

23. Davila J, Mattson WW, O'Neill TJE et al. A method for surgical correction of mitral insufficiency. Surg Gynecol Obstet 1954; 98:407-12.

24. Glover RP, Henderson AR, Marguitti R et al. The fate of intracardiac pericardial grafts as applied to the closure of septal defects and its relief of mitral insufficiency. Surgical Forum 1953; 3:178-85.

25. Jorden P, Wible J. A spring valve for mitral insufficiency. Arch Surg 1955; 71:468-74.

26. Bakst AA, Boley SJ, Edward J et al. The surgical correction of mitral insufficiency by the use of pericardial grafts. J Thorac Surg 1958; 35:492-502.

27. Moore TC, Shumacker HB. The unsuitability of atrioventricular autogenous slings for diminishing valvular insufficiency. Surgery 1953; 33:173-82.

28. Henderson AR, Law CL. The surgical treatment of mitral insufficiency. Surgery 1953; 33:858-68.

29. DeWall RA, Warden HE, Lillehei CW et al. A prosthesis for the palliation of mitral insufficiency. Dis Chest 1956; 30:133-40.

30. Johns TNP, Blalock A. Mitral insufficiency: The experimental use of a mobile polyvinyl sponge prosthesis. Ann Surg 1954; 140:335-41.

31. Harken DE, Black H, Ellis LB et al. The surgical correction of mitral insufficiency. J Thorac Surg 1954; 28:604-27.

32. Glenn WWL, Gentsch TO, Hume M et al. The surgical treatment of mitral insufficiency with particular reference to the application of a vertically suspended graft. Surgery 1956; 40:59-77.

33. Kay EB, Nogueira C, Head LR et al. Surgical treatment of mitral insufficiency. J Thorac Surg 1958; 36:677-96.

34. Lillehei CW, Gott VL, DeWall RA et al. The surgical treatment of stenotic or regurgitant lesions of the mitral and aortic valves by direct vision utilizing a pump oxygenator. J Thorac Surg 1958; 35:154-90.

35. Barnard CN, Schrire U. Ivalon baffle for posterior leaflet replacement in the treatment of mitral insufficiency: A follow-up study. Surgery 1968; 63:727-30.

36. Orszulak TA, Schaff HV, Danielson GK et al. Mitral regurgitation due to ruptured chordae tendineae. J Thorac Cardiovasc Surg 1985; 89:491-8.

37. McGoon DC. Repair of mitral insufficiency due to ruptured chordae tendineae. J Thorac Cardiovasc Surg 1960; 39:357-62.

38. McGoon DC. An early approach to the repair of ruptured mitral chordae. Ann Thorac

Surg 1989; 47:628-9.

39. Sauvage LR, Gross RE, Rudolph AM et al. Experimental study of tissue and prosthetic grafts with selected application to clinical intracardiac surgery. Ann Surg 1961; 153:321-43.

40. Sauvage LR, Wood SJ, Bill Jr AH. Pericardial autografts in the mitral valve. A preliminary report. J Thorac Cardiovasc Surg 1962; 44:67-72.

41. Frater RWM, Berghuis J, Brown A et al. The use of autogenous pericardium for posterior mitral leaflet replacement: An experimental and clinical study. Surgery 1963; 54:260-8.

42. Frater RWM. Anatomical rules for plastic repair of the diseased mitral valve. Thorax 1964; 19:458-64.

43. Frater RWM, Berghuis J, Brown AL et al. The experimental and clinical use of autogenous pericardium for the replacement and extension of mitral and tricuspid valve cusps and chordae. J Cardiovasc Surg (Torino) 1965; 6:214-28.

44. Carpentier A, Lemaigre G, Robert L et al. Biological factors affecting long-term results in valvular heterografts. J Thorac Cardiovasc Surg 1969; 58:467-83.

45. Carpentier A. La valvuloplastie reconstitutive. Une nouvelle techniques de valvuloplastie mitrale. Presse Med. 1969; 77:251-3.

46. Carpentier A, Deloche A, Dauptain J et al. A new reconstructive operation for correction of mitral and tricuspid insufficiency. J Thorac Cardiovasc Surg 1971; 61:1-13.

47. Carpentier A, Relland J, Deloche A et al. Conservative management of the prolapsed mitral valve. Ann Thorac Surg 1978; 26:294-302.

48. Carpentier A, Chauvaud S, Fabiani JN et al. Reconstructive surgery of mitral incompetence. Ten-year appraisal. J Thorac Cardiovasc Surg 1980; 79:338-48.

49. Carpentier A. Cardiac valve surgery—The "French correction." J Thorac Cardiovasc Surg 1983; 86:323-37.

50. Deloche A, Jebara VA, Relland JYM et al. Valve repair with Carpentier techniques. The second decade. J Thorac Cardiovasc Surg 1990; 99:990-1002.

51. Dreyfus G, Serraf A, Jebara VA et al. Valve repair in acute endocarditis. Ann Thorac Surg 1990; 49:706-13.

52. Chauvaud S, Jebara V, Chachques JC et al. Valve extension with glutaraldehyde-preserved autologous pericardium. Results in mitral valve repair. J Thorac Cardiovasc Surg 1991; 102:171-8.

53. Cosgrove DM. Mitral valve repair in patients with elongated chordae tendineae. J Cardiac Surg 1989; 4:247-52.

54. Kreindel MS, Schiavone WA, Lever HM et al. Systolic anterior motion of the mitral valve after Carpentier ring valvuloplasty for mitral valve prolapse. Am J Cardiol 1986; 57:408-12.

55. Carpentier A. The S.A.M. issue. "Le Club Mitrale" Newsletter. 1989; 1:5.

56. Carpentier A. The sliding leaflet technique. "Le Club Mitrale" Newsletter 1988; 1:5.

57. Yacoub M, Halim M, Radley-Smith R et al. Surgical treatment of mitral regurgitation caused by floppy valves: Repair versus replacement. Circulation 1981; 64 (Suppl II):II 210-II 216.

58. Frater RWM. Mitral valve anatomy and prosthetic valve design. Proceedings Staff Meeting Mayo Clin. 1961; 36:582-92.

59. Frater RWM, Gabbay S, Shore D et al. Reproducible replacement of elongated or ruptured mitral valve chordae. Ann Thorac Surg 1983; 35:14-28.

60. Frater RWM. Functional anatomy of the mitral valve. In: Ionescu MI, Cohn LH, eds. Mitral valve disease: Diagnosis and treatment. London: Butterworths, 1985:127-38.

61. Shore DF, Gabbay S, Yellin EL et al. Degenerative changes in glutaraldehyde-preserved pericardium used for the experimental replacement of anterior chordae of the mitral valve. J Cardiovasc Surg 1983; 24:132-7.

62. Gabbay S, Bortolotti U, Factor S et al. Calcification of implanted xenograft pericardium. Influence of site and function. J Thorac Cardiovasc Surg 1984; 87:782-7.

63. Bortolotti U, Gallo JI, Gabbay S et al. Replacement of mitral valve chordae with autologous pericardium in dogs. Thorac Cardiovasc Surgeon 1984; 32:15-7.

64. Bortolotti U, Zussa C, Factor S et al. Glutaraldehyde treated auto, homo and xenograft pericardium in atrial, mitral, aortic

and pericardial applications. Life Support Systems 1986; 4:148-50.

65. Vetter HO, Factor SM, Frater RWM. The use of glycerol-treated homologous pericardium as a substitute for cusps and chordae tendineae of the mitral valve in sheep. Thorac Cardiovasc Surgeon 1987; 35:11-5.

66. Frater RWM. Discussion of: Chauvaud S, Jebara V, Chachques JC et al. Valve extension with glutaraldehyde-preserved autologous pericardium. Results in mitral valve repair. J Thorac Cardiovasc Surg 1991; 102:171-8.

67. Sauvage LR, Wood SJ. Techique for correction of mitral insufficiency by leaflet advancement. J Thorac Cardiovasc Surg 1966; 51:649-57.

68. Holdefer WF, Edwards S, Dowling ER. An experimental approach to mitral valve replacement with autologous pericardium. J Thorac Cardiovasc Surg 1968; 55:873-81.

69. Cleland WP. Pericardial repair of the mitral valve. In: Ionescu MI, Ross DN, Wooler GH, eds. Biological tissue in heart valve replacement. London: Butterworth, 1972: 703-7.

70. Flege J, Rossi N, Auer J et al. Mitral valve replacement with autologous fascia lata. Surg Forum 1967; 18:116-20.

71. Gilbert J, Mansour K, Sanders S et al. Experimental reconstruction of the tricuspid valve with autologous fascia lata. Arch Surg 1968; 97:149-53.

72. Ionescu MI, Deac R, Whitaker W et al. Fascia lata heart valves in biological tissue in heart valve replacement. In: Ionescu MI, Ross DN, Wooler GH, eds. Biological tissue in heart valve replacement. London: Butterworth, 1972:617-85.

73. Bodnar E. Discussion of: Chauvaud S, Jebara V, Chachques JC et al. Valve extension with glutaraldehyde-preserved autologous pericardium. Results in mitral valve repair. J Thorac Cardiovasc Surg 1991; 102:171-8.

74. Hisatomi K, Isomura T, Hirano A et al. Long-term follow-up results after reconstruction of the mitral valve by leaflet advancement. Ann Thorac Surg 1992; 54:271-5.

75. Duran CG, Pomar JL, Revuelta JM et al. Conservative operation for mitral insufficiency. Critical analysis supported by postoperative hemodynamic studies of 72 patients. J

Thorac Cardiovasc Surg 1980; 79:326-37.

76. Duran CMG, Ubago JL. Conservative mitral valve surgery. Problems and developments in the techniques of prosthetic ring annuloplasty. In: Kalmanson D, ed. The mitral valve. A pluridisciplinary approach. Acton, Mass: Publishing Sciences Group Inc, 1975:549-57.

77. Duran CG. Surgical management of elongated chordae of the mitral valve. J Cardiac Surg 1989; 4:253-9.

78. Cosgrove DM. Surgery for degenerative mitral valve disease. Semin Thorac Cardiovasc Surg 1989; 1:183-93.

79. Jebara VA, Dervanian P, Acar C et al. Mitral valve repair using Carpentier techniques in patients more than 70 years old. Early and late results. Circulation 1992; 86 (Suppl II):II 53-II 59.

80. Hvass U, Pansard Y, Lamberti A et al. Reparation de lesions mitrales rhumatismales par transfert d'un segment de la valve posterieure avec ses cordages sur la valve anterieure. Arch Mal Coeur 1986; 79:103-6.

81. Lessana A, Romano M, Lutfalla G et al. Treatment of ruptured or elongated anterior mitral valve chordae by partial transposition of the posterior leaflet: Experience with 29 patients. Ann Thorac Surg 1988; 45:404-8.

82. Gregory Jr F, Takeda R, Silva S et al. A new technique for repair of mitral insufficiency caused by ruptured chordae of the anterior leaflet. J Thorac Cardiovasc Surg 1988; 96:765-8.

83. Sutlic Z, Schmid C, Borst HG. Repair of flail anterior leaflets of tricuspid and mitral valves by cusp remodeling. Ann Thorac Surg 1990; 50:927-30.

84. Koutlas TC, deBruijn NP, Sheikh KH et al. Chordal rupture as a late complication after mitral valve reconstruction. J Thorac Cardiovasc Surg 1991; 102:466-8.

85. Jebara VA, Acar C, Deloche A. Tricuspid and mitral valve repair. Ann Thorac Surg 1991; 52:896-900.

86. Acar J, Caramanian M, Perrault M. Les insuffisances mitrales par rupture de cordages. Arch Mal Coeur 1968; 61:17-24.

87. Lessana A, Escorsin M, Romano M et al. Transposition of posterior leaflet for treat-

ment of ruptured main chordae of the anterior mitral leaflet. J Thorac Cardiovasc Surg 1985; 89:804-6.

88. Lessana A, Tran Viet T, Ades F et al. Mitral reconstructive operations: A series of 130 consecutive cases. J Thorac Cardiovasc Surg 1983; 86:553-61.

89. Frater RWM. Discussion of: Lessana A, Romano M, Lutfalla G et al. Treatment of ruptured or elongated anterior mitral valve chordae by partial transposition of the posterior leaflet: Experience with 29 patients. Ann Thorac Surg 1988; 45:404-8.

90. David TE. Discussion of: Lessana A, Romano

M, Lutfalla G et al. Treatment of ruptured or elongated anterior mitral valve chordae by partial transposition of the posterior leaflet: Experience with 29 patients. Ann Thorac Surg 1988; 45:404-8.

91. Colvin SB. Discussion of: Lessana A, Romano M, Lutfalla G et al. Treatment of ruptured or elongated anterior mitral valve chordae by partial transposition of the posterior leaflet: Experience with 29 patients. Ann Thorac Surg 1988; 45:404-8.

92. Alvarez JM, Teoh N, Deal CW. Repairing the degenerative anterior mitral leaflet. Ann Thorac Surg 1992; 54:1229-30.

CHAPTER 5

CHORDAL REPLACEMENT

Many different techniques have been proposed and clinically tested to correct mitral valve dysfunctions produced by chordal alterations. In cases of chordal fusion, fenestration associated with commissurotomy and papillary muscle splitting improves diastolic motion of the leaflets reducing resistance to blood flow. When secondary chordae are retracted they can be dissected without any significant weakening of leaflet support.[1] If leaflet excursion is excessive due to chordal elongation or rupture different methods of chordal shortening (invagination into papillary muscle, looping at the papillary or leaflet side, papillary muscle head repositioning), rectangular resection of the posterior leaflet, chordae transposition, and sliding procedures are practicable. However it is common for outstanding cardiac surgeons to encounter cases in which the application of these traditional procedures are not feasible or will not enhance late results.

Before introducing posterior chordae transposition to the anterior leaflet, Carpentier considered that valve repair was contraindicated if more than 25% of the anterior leaflet must be plicated or resected.[2] In 1980, reviewing his ten-year experience with mitral valve reconstruction, he defined indications and contraindications for this operation.[3] The relative indications included: ruptured chordae of more than one-third and less than one-half of the posterior leaflet, rupture of a paramedian chorda of the anterior leaflet, elongated chordae of more than one-third of the mural leaflet, or elongation of anterior leaflet chordae. Contraindications included ruptured chordae of more than one-half the posterior leaflet or rupture of a main chorda of the anterior leaflet. Carpentier also stressed that chordal shortening is a difficult, time consuming procedure, requiring intensive training.

Similar restrictions in indications for valve repair have been reported by Orszulak et al from the Mayo Clinic.[4] In particular they were reluctant to repair a valve when a ruptured main anterior chorda was associated with weak adjacent chordae. With their technique of leaflet plication they realized that this method is not appropriate when a significant plication of the anterior leaflet is required because this maneuver can cause tissue stretching with consequent commissural regurgitation. Other authors were reluctant to perform valve repair when the anterior leaflet was involved in the mechanism of regurgitation.[5-7]

Similar concern was expressed by Frater[8] and Duran.[9] In the event of anterior chordae rupture Duran preferred to replace the valve, whereas Frater suggested chordal replacement. In two recent papers Craver[10] and Kaul[11] and co-workers reported their criteria of exclusion from valve repair. Craver included severe fibroelastic deficiency, irreparable rheumatic lesions, and extensive endocardial necrosis due to myocardial infarction. In addition to extensive fibroelastic tissue deficiency, Kaul included also degeneration of more than 25% of a leaflet and rupture of central chordae. In any case, the fate of elongated chordae, once they are shortened, and that of adjacent chordae is still not known.

Although some authors[8,12,13] assume that stress is distributed among all chordae minimizing the probability of further chordal rupture, in cases of successfully repaired degenerative mitral incompetence, other clinical series report rupture. Koutlas[14] described three cases of chordal rupture less than one year after having been shortened. The author suggested two possible mechanisms are responsible for this complication: excessive stress placed on the weakened, shortened chorda, or a sawing effect of the suture utilized to bend and shorten this chorda. Orszulak,[4] reporting the Mayo Clinic experience in mitral valve repair, described the rupture of chordae not involved in the first operation, as one of the complications, produced by progression of the degenerative pathology, requiring reoperation. Reviewing his experience with chordal replacement with

pericardium, Frater, in 1983, affirmed that restoration of competence, as a result of valve repair, may reduce the stress on remaining natural chordae, thereby explaining the absence of further chordal rupture.[8] Nevertheless seven years later, reporting the long-term follow-up of the same group of 18 patients, he described the need for reoperation in one case, due to chordal rupture of the lateral half of the anterior cusp, while at first operation the broken chordae of the medial half of the same leaflet had been replaced with pericardial grafts.[15]

CHORDAL REPLACEMENT WITH BIOLOGICAL MATERIALS

All of these supposed contraindications and incompletely solved situations compelled some researchers to investigate the feasibility of chordal replacement, the most obvious solution in cases of extensive chordal pathology.

Duran[13] and Cosgrove,[16] considering all the possible options available to treat chordal pathology, suggested artificial chordal utilization as a field to explore for selected situations, although clinical experience was still too limited (Fig. 5.1). This operation was described in some reports 30 years ago.[17-21] Different kinds of suture—nylon, silk,

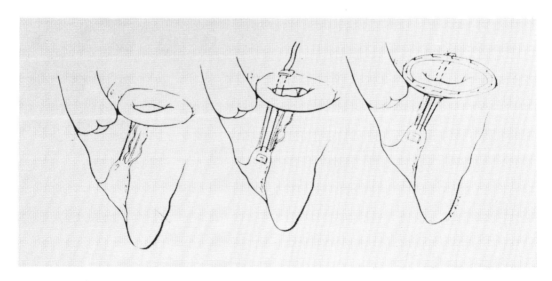

Fig. 5.1. Chordal replacement with sutures, proposed in cases of anterior chordal pathology. (From CG Duran. Surgical management of elongated chordae of the mitral valve. J Cardiac Surg 1989; 4:253-9. Reproduced with permission of the author and Futura Publishing Co, Inc.).

teflon—were utilized to replace mostly posterior chordae. The results were uneven.

As mentioned in the chapter on mitral valve repair, during the same period Frater et al tested biological materials, such as fresh autologous pericardium, to replace leaflet and chordae (Fig. 4.5 and 4.6 of Chapter 4) with unsatisfactory results, for the stiffening and shrinking of pericardial implants.[22-25]

Different behavior was observed with the same material by Rittenhouse and co-workers[26] who reported satisfactory results after up to nine years of follow-up. The greatest improvement was produced by tanning procedures with glutaraldehyde. The utilization of glutaraldehyde-tanned xenograft pericardium for chordal replacement yielded acceptable long-term results, although in small series of patients from Frater et al.[15] An interesting observation was reported in this paper. One patient had received the simultaneous replacement of ruptured chordae of the anterior leaflet, with strips of xenograft glutaraldehyde treated pericardium, and of a calcific aortic valve, with a bioprosthesis made with the same material, obtained from the same manufacturer. Eight years later the aortic bioprosthesis was replaced for massive calcification, while artificial chordae were still functional, without apparent signs of calcification. This observation validates previous experimental findings that the site of implantation and the different stress load greatly influence material behavior.[27,28]

From the positive experience with glutaraldehyde-tanned xenograft pericardium in chordal position, Frater[8] drew some conclusions in order to delineate the limits of this technique. He stated that it is reasonable to utilize pericardial chordae when less than half of the valve has elongated or ruptured chordae. This statement was substantiated by the observation that, after a long follow-up, a valve can retain satisfactory function in the presence of one stiff, non-pliable pericardial chorda, provided all other chordae are normally pliable. On the other hand subvalvular apparatus pathology often involves many groups of chordae of both leaflets therefore limiting utilization of pericardial chordal replacement.

CHORDAL REPLACEMENT WITH ARTIFICIAL MATERIALS

Seeking a better substitute for mitral chordae when traditional procedures were not adequate, to the best of our knowledge from the literature, in the mid-80s, three independent research groups evaluated a new suture to be utilized in this site.

Expanded-polytetrafluoroethylene (e-PTFE) was simultaneously tested at the University of Toronto and the Toronto Hospital (Canada),[29] at the Hospital Nacional Marques de Valdecilla, Santander (Spain),[30] and at the Albert Einstein College of Medicine, Bronx, NY (U.S.A.).[31,32] This suture, called Gore-Tex®, is produced by W.L. Gore & Associates, Inc., Flagstaff, AZ, U.S.A. It is manufactured entirely from a single strand of PTFE that has been expanded to form a porous microstructure (Fig. 5.2). It is composed of solid nodes and connecting, oriented fibrils of PTFE (Fig. 5.3), producing a network, and contains more than 50% air by volume.[31]

This microstructure allows infiltration of tissue cells (fibroblasts and leukocytes) producing firm tissue adherence and collagen fibers penetration. PTFE is one of the most inert materials. It is not subject to hydrolysis or other chemical degradation in vivo, nor is it weakened by tissue or bacterial enzymes. On the contrary, host tissue adhesion and infiltration increase suture strength with time.

These properties have been described in an independent recent study of Cochran and Kunzelman[33] who compared Gore-Tex® and braided polyester sutures with fresh porcine mitral chordae. They evaluated the viscoelastic properties of these materials and found that e-PTFE is the substitute that most closely shares natural chordal characteristics, while braided polyester failed to show any viscoelastic behavior, suggesting the potential for fatigue and failure. e-PTFE has some degree of hysteresis, since under controlled loading-unloading cycles it doesn't recover completely from the strain. This phenomenon is more pronounced after the first cycle and then decreases significantly; eventually it recovers almost completely from any further strain. The extent of this phenomenon is about 1.1%, in an experimental model. This "creep" (elongation) could represent a long-term problem, but the evidence of tissue incorporation suggests increased viscoelasticity and strength with time.[33]

The characteristics and the consequent theoretical advantages of this material stimulated our interest to study the possible utilization of e-PTFE for chordal replacement. The following chapters will describe our experience with this type of material both in experimental and clinical settings.

REFERENCES

1. Kunzelman KS, Cochran RP. Mechanical properties of basal and marginal mitral valve chordae tendineae. ASAIO Trans 1990; 36:M 405-8.
2. Carpentier A, Deloche A, Dauptain J et al. A new reconstructive operation for correction of mitral and tricuspid insufficiency. J Thorac Cardiovasc Surg 1971; 61:1-13.
3. Carpentier A, Chauvaud S, Fabiani JN et al. Reconstructive surgery of mitral incompetence. Ten-year appraisal. J Thorac Cardiovasc Surg 1980; 79:338-48.
4. Orszulak TA, Schaff HV, Danielson GK et al. Mitral regurgitation due to ruptured chordae tendineae. J Thorac Cardiovasc Surg 1985; 89:491-8.
5. Messmer BJ, Gattiker K, Rothlin M et al. Reconstruction of the mitral valve. Ann Thorac Surg 1973; 16:30-43.
6. Ross BA, Fox C, Hedley BA et al. Late results of valvuloplasty for mitral regurgitation due to rupture of chordae of the posterior (mural) cusp. J Thorac Cardiovasc Surg 1971; 71:533-6.
7. West PN, Weldon CS. Reconstructive valve surgery. Ann Thorac Surg 1978; 25:167-77.
8. Frater RWM, Gabbay S, Shore D et al. Reproducible replacement of elongated or ruptured mitral valve chordae. Ann Thorac Surg 1983; 35:14-28.
9. Duran CG. Discussion of: Frater RWM, Gabbay S, Shore D et al: Reproducible replacement of elongated or ruptured mitral valve chordae. Ann Thorac Surg 1983; 35:14-28.

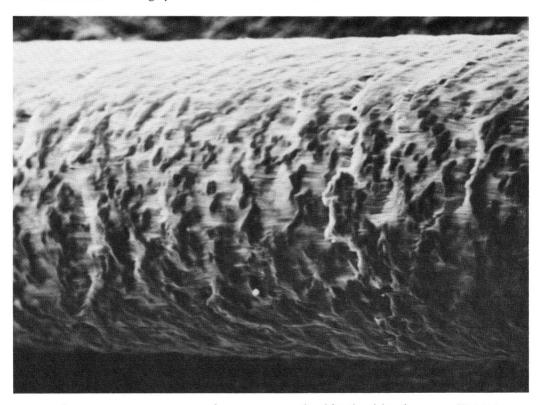

Fig. 5.2. Characteristic porous structure of e-PTFE sutures utilized for chordal replacement. SEM 176x.

10. Craver JM, Cohen C, Weintraub WS. Case-matched comparison of mitral valve replacement and repair. Ann Thorac Surg 1990; 49:964-9.

11. Kaul TK, Ramsdale DR, Meek D et al. Mitral valve replacement in patients with severe mitral regurgitation and impaired left ventricular function. Int J Cardiol 1992; 35:169-79.

12. Gregory Jr F, Takeda R, Silva S et al. A new technique for repair of mitral insufficiency caused by ruptured chordae of the anterior leaflet. J Thorac Cardiovasc Surg 1988; 96:765-8.

13. Duran CG. Surgical management of elongated chordae of the mitral valve. J Cardiac Surg 1989; 4:253-9.

14. Koutlas TC, deBruijn NP, Sheikh KH et al. Chordal rupture as a late complication after mitral valve reconstruction. J Thorac Cardiovasc Surg 1991; 102:466-8.

15. Frater RWM, Vetter HO, Zussa C et al. Chordal replacement in mitral valve repair. Circulation 1990; 82 (Suppl IV):IV 125-IV 130.

16. Cosgrove DM. Mitral valve repair in patients with elongated chordae tendineae. J Cardiac Surg 1989; 4:247-52.

17. January LE, Fisher JM, Ehrenhalf J. Mitral insufficiency resulting from rupture of normal chordae tendineae. Circulation 1962; 26:1329-33.

18. Morris JD, Penner DA, Brandt RL. Surgical correction of ruptured chordae tendineae. J Thorac Cardiovasc Surg 1964; 48:772-80.

19. Sanders CA, Scannell JG, Harthorne JW et al. Severe mitral regurgitation secondary to ruptured chordae tendineae. Circulation 1965; 31:506-16.

20. Kay JH, Tsuji HK, Redington JV. The surgical treatment of mitral insufficiency associated with torn chordae tendineae. Ann Thorac Surg 1965; 1:269-76.

21. Marchand P, Barlow JB, Du Plessis LA et al. Mitral regurgitation with rupture of normal chordae tendineae. Br Heart J 1966; 28:746-58.

22. Frater RWM. Mitral valve anatomy and prosthetic valve design. Proc Staff Mtg Mayo Clin 1961; 36:582-92.

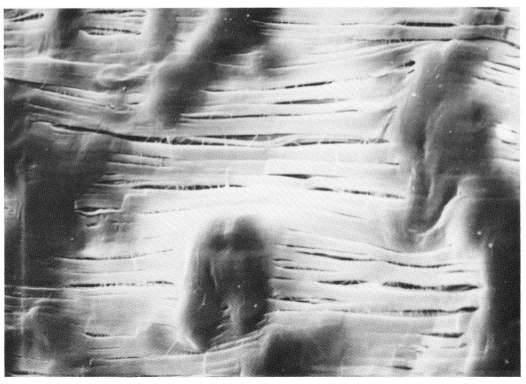

Fig. 5.3. At higher magnification solid nodes and connecting oriented fibrils of PTFE are evident. The structure contains more than 50% air by volume and should allow infiltration by host tissue. SEM 1460x.

23. Frater RWM, Berghuis J, Brown A et al. The use of autogenous pericardium for posterior mitral leaflet replacement: An experimental and clinical study. Surgery 1963; 54:260-8.

24. Frater RWM. Anatomical rules for plastic repair of the diseased mitral valve. Thorax 1964; 19:458-64.

25. Frater RWM, Berghuis J, Brown AL et al. The experimental and clinical use of autogenous pericardium for the replacement and extension of mitral and tricuspid valve cusps and chordae. J Cardiovasc Surg (Torino) 1965; 6:214-28.

26. Rittenhouse EA, Davis CC, Wood SJ et al. Replacement of ruptured chordae tendineae of the mitral valve with autologous pericardial chordae. J Thorac Cardiovasc Surg 1978; 75:870-6.

27. Hvass U, Pansard Y, Lamberti A et al. Reparation de lesions mitrales rhumatismales par transfert d'un segment de la valve posterieure avec ses cordages sur la valve anterieure. Arch Mal Coeur 1986; 79:103-6.

28. Bortolotti U, Zussa C, Factor S et al. Glutaraldehyde treated auto, homo and xenograft pericardium in atrial, mitral, aortic and pericardial applications. Life Support Systems 1986; 4:148-50.

29. David TE. Discussion of: Lessana A, Romano M, Lutfalla G et al. Treatment of ruptured or elongated anterior mitral valve chordae by partial transposition of the posterior leaflet: Experience with 29 patients. Ann Thorac Surg 1988; 45:404-8.

30. Revuelta JM, Garcia-Rinaldi R, Gaite L et al. Generation of chordae tendineae with polytetrafluoroethylene stents. Results of mitral valve chordal replacement in sheep. J Thorac Cardiovasc Surg 1989; 97:98-103.

31. Vetter HO, Burack JH, Factor SM et al. Replacement of chordae tendineae of the mitral valve using the new expanded PTFE suture in sheep. In: Bodnar E, Yacoub M, eds. Biologic and bioprosthetic valves. New York: Yorke Medical Books, 1986:772-84.

32. Zussa C, Frater RWM, Galloni SM et al. Expanded polytetrafluoroethylene as mitral valve chordae substitute. Proceedings of third world biomaterials congress. Kyoto, Japan, April 21-25,1988:128.

33. Cochran RP, Kunzelman KS. Comparison of viscoelastic properties of suture versus porcine mitral valve chordae tendineae. J Card Surg 1991; 6:508-13.

CHAPTER 6

ARTIFICIAL CHORDAE—ANIMAL EXPERIMENTS

In 1984 Vetter and co-workers started animal experiments at Albert Einstein College of Medicine, Bronx, NY, utilizing 2-0 and 3-0 Gore-Tex® sutures in a sheep model. The experiments were designed to answer a series of questions, summarized by Vetter in his report:[1] essentially whether artificial chordae could successfully replace anterior leaflet chordae, healing at both papillary muscle and leaflet sides. The incidence of thromboembolism and the long-term fate of these chordal substitutes were evaluated as well.

The authors sacrificed the animals after hemodynamic study and M-mode echocardiography to verify mitral valve competence at different times after operation to recognize possible time-related artificial chordae behavior variations. All specimens showed good healing of artificial chordae to the host tissue. A fibrous sheath covered artificial chordae as a self-limiting process, since it was present by four months after operation and seemed not to increase with time (9 and 12 months specimens). No thrombi or platelet accumulations could be detected, nor did calcifications appear on X-ray examination. Anticipated host tissue adhesion occurred by collagen fibers infiltration of internodal spaces. The final diameter of the neo-chordae was greater than natural chordae, although this factor did not seem to interfere with valve function.

The experimental design was limited, since only a couple of artificial chordae had been utilized and consequently their thickening was counterbalanced by the normal flexibility of all the remaining natural chordae.

The encouraging results of these experiments encouraged our group to test thinner Gore-Tex® sutures in the chordal position to evaluate whether these would generate artificial chordae with diameter and flexibility similar to natural chordae. If this were possible, we might utilize many artificial chordae in particularly complicated valve repair.

In the Cardiovascular Research Laboratory of the same Institution, in 1985 we performed eight additional animal experiments. Dogs (naturally hypertensive greyhounds) were utilized in four cases, while weanling sheep were used in the others. Hypertensive dogs were chosen to evaluate any possible influence of high closure pressure of the mitral valve on long-term artificial chordae behavior, particularly with regard to "fatigue" and "creep" phenomena. All animals received humane care in compliance with the "Guide for Care and Use of Laboratory Animals" published by the National Institutes of Health (NIH publication No. 85-23, revised 1985).

Mean body weight was 27.2+/-0.3 kg for dogs and 29.3+/-4.2 kg for sheep.

Sheep were sheared the day before operation and all animals were fasted for 24 hours.

SURGICAL TECHNIQUE

Anesthesia was induced with 2 mg/kg thiopental sodium and maintained with halothane after orotracheal intubation and mechanical ventilation. In dogs, the left femoral artery was cannulated for arterial pressure monitoring and blood gas sampling, while in sheep these parameters were obtained from a derivation of the arterial line for cardiopulmonary bypass.

The heart was exposed by left thoracotomy through the fourth intercostal space. After heparin administration (1.5 mg/kg),

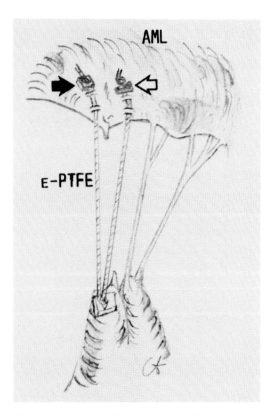

Fig. 6.1. Schematic illustration of artificial chordae (e-PTFE) insertion in animals. On the leaflet side one strand is fixed over a PTFE pledget (black arrow), while the other is fixed over a hemoclip (empty arrow). AML=anterior mitral leaflet.

cannulation of right (dogs) or left (sheep) femoral artery was performed for systemic arterial perfusion from cardiopulmonary bypass, while venous return was obtained cannulating the right atrial appendage. In normothermic cardiopulmonary bypass and beating heart, the left atrium was opened through a longitudinal incision from the tip of the atrial appendage to the left pulmonary veins.

In one dog artificial chordae were added to natural chordae, while in the other animals two to four marginal chordae of the anterior leaflet were resected and replaced. Double-armed 5-0 Gore-Tex® sutures were brought through the fibrous tip of the papillary muscle in the place of emergence of resected chordae (Fig. 6.1). They were fixed in mattress shape, reinforcing on both sides of the muscle with Teflon or PTFE pledgets, and tied. The two arms of each suture were then connected separately to the unsupported area of the anterior leaflet. The strands were brought twice through the leaflet 2 mm apart starting from the ventricular surface of the free edge. The proper length of the artificial chordae was set in such a way that the free margins of the opposite leaflets hung at the same level into the ventricle in each corresponding area.[2-4] Finally each arm of the suture was fixed separately, tying around either a hemostatic clip (Edward Weck, Research Triangle Park, NC, U.S.A.), utilized also to keep the set length, or a small Gore-Tex® pledget (Fig. 6.1). The left atrium was then closed, leaving a small catheter inside to record left atrial pressure. A catheter was also inserted through the free wall into left ventricle.

The animals were then weaned from cardiopulmonary bypass. Venous and arterial cannulae were removed, and protamine sulfate (1.5 mg/kg) was administered, adjusting the dosage on the basis of activated coagulation time control. The average cardiopulmonary bypass time was 27.5 ±4.3 minutes. Left atrial and left ventricular pressures were simultaneously recorded to evaluate the presence of mitral stenosis or incompetence. One gram cephalothin was given immediately before and after surgery and then once a day for five days. No anticoagulant regimen was instituted.

INTRAOPERATIVE RESULTS

Transvalvular gradients were detected in none of the animals. A "v" wave suggestive of mild mitral incompetence was recorded in one dog. All animals awakened from anesthesia and were examined for heart murmurs. The dog, intraoperatively showing a "v" wave, manifested a 3/6 systolic murmur, without evident signs of hemodynamic impairment. Another dog bled significantly into the chest drainage and hematological tests disclosed a coagulopathy that could not be reversed. The animal died 24 hours after operation. All other animals recovered and were available for follow-up.

FOLLOW-UP

The seven surviving animals were checked by the physician for signs of mitral incompetence or heart failure every day for the first month and then once a week. Except for the dog with 3/6 murmur since the operation—which had stable auscultatory findings and no signs of heart failure—no other manifestations of mitral regurgitation could be detected in any animal for the entire follow-up period. They were electively sacrificed 6 to 13 months after operation.

The average body weight of sheep at sacrifice was 39.2 ±3.7 kg, while dogs showed no significant differences from the weight at operation. Before sacrifice, cardiac catheterization and left ventriculography were performed. Seven animals were available for these examinations and hemodynamic data were collected in basal anesthetized condition and under pressure load obtained with administration of 1 μg/kg/min of epinephrine (Table 6.1). The hearts were then carefully examined for presence of thrombi, and gross examination of mitral valve apparatus was performed to evidence calcifications, tears, suture dehiscence. Also a hydrodynamic test of valve competence was performed.

A few artificial chordae were utilized for testing flexibility, while all other specimens were fixed in 10% formaldehyde for light microscopy, or in buffered glutaraldehyde and then dehydrated and gold-palladium coated for scanning electron microscopy (SEM). The same specimens were subsequently utilized for transmission electron microscopy (TEM).

HEMODYNAMIC DATA

Cardiac catheterization was performed with the animals anesthetized with thiopental sodium and without utilization of any anesthetic gas. Data were acquired in closed chest situation at basal conditions and under different inotropic situations.

In basal conditions mean left atrial pressure in dogs was 6.7 mmHg, in sheep it was 4.5 mmHg. In one dog a "v" wave of 12 mmHg was present (at operation, early after weaning from cardiopulmonary bypass, it was 14 mmHg). Systolic left ventricular pressures were 158.3 mmHg, and 115 mmHg, in dogs and sheep, respectively. Heart rate was 124 beats/min in dogs, and 96.2 beats/min in sheep.

During infusion of epinephrine 1 μg/kg/min heart rate rose to 174 beats/min in dogs, and 128.2 beats/min in sheep, while atrial pressures were respectively 9.3 mmHg and 6 mmHg. The dog with mild mitral regurgitation showed a "v" wave increased to 18 mmHg. Ventricular pressure increased to 215 mmHg in dogs and to 152.5 mmHg in sheep. Left ventriculography revealed 2+ mitral regurgitation only in the dog with the "v" wave and known systolic murmur since operation.

GROSS EXAMINATION

Liver and kidneys were always examined for signs of thromboembolism. None was detected.

A thrombus, the size of a bean, was found in the left atrium of a dog, at the site where the atrial retractor was placed for operation. In the same area and along the atriotomy suture line calcifications were noted. No other thrombi or calcifications were detected in any heart.

Incorrect artificial chordae length at operation was associated with a tear in the anterolateral commissural tissue. This was discovered to be the cause of the moderate regurgitation reported in a dog since operation.

In a sheep the two ends of the same Gore-Tex® suture had been placed too close. This caused them to fuse (Fig. 6.2), being incorporated into a single fibrous sheath (Fig. 6.3). The resultant structure, although stiffer

Table 1. Hemodynamic results after artificial chordae insertion before animal sacrifice

Animal	#	Months	LAP	LVSP	HR	Regurg
BASAL						
d	1	6	4	170	125	No
d	2	12	9 (v 12)	145	136	Moderate
d	3	13	7	160	112	No
Mean			6.7	158.3	124	
s	1	6	5	100	90	No
s	2	9	6	110	110	No
s	3	12	2	135	85	No
s	4	13	5	115	100	No
Mean			4.5	115	96.2	
EPINEPHRINE						
d	1	6	7	230	175	No
d	2	12	12 (v 18)	195	182	Moderate
d	3	13	9	220	165	No
Mean			9.3	215	174	
s	1	6	6	165	120	No
s	2	9	6	150	118	No
s	3	12	5	150	130	No
s	4	13	7	145	145	No
Mean			6	152.5	128.2	

Months=months from operation; LAP=left atrial pressure (mm Hg); LVSP=left ventricular systolic pressure (mm Hg); HR=heart rate (beats/min); regurg=mitral regurgitation at left ventriculography; d=dog; s=sheep

than natural chordae, was only slightly thicker (Fig. 6.4).

Healing to the papillary muscle was good in all specimens with almost complete disappearance of pledgets, covered by smooth fibrous tissue overgrowth. On the leaflet side a mild inflammatory reaction was evident in one sheep and one dog. It was probably related to the presence of the hemoclip and produced minor retraction of the free edge of the leaflet, without any hemodynamic relevance (Fig. 6.5).

Three fresh artificial chordae were utilized to compare their flexibility with that of natural chordae, just by simple observation. They were retrieved from animals sacrificed at different intervals after operation. An artificial chorda and a natural chorda cut at the same length were suspended by one end and left hanging by gravity on a scaled paper to evaluate the degree of bending (Fig. 6.6). We could not find any significant difference, even in the

case of an artificial chordae retrieved 13 months after operation.[5]

Macroscopic examination of artificial chordae revealed diameters quite similar to natural chordae only after fibrous sheath overgrowth (Fig. 6.7), while, before this process was complete, Gore-Tex® sutures were thinner than natural chordae (Fig. 6.8). The six-month specimens appeared incompletely covered in the centrally, while after seven months one animal had a fibrous sheath extending from the pledgets utilized on the papillary muscle to the cusp attachment. Chordae with a longer follow-up didn't exhibit a greater thickness of their sheath, having a final diameter comparable to that of sutures with a shorter period of implantation (Fig. 6.9).

These observations confirmed Vetter's findings[1] and suggested the self-limiting character of this type of fibrous tissue overgrowth. Except for the dog with an incorrect artificial chordae measurement at operation, all speci-

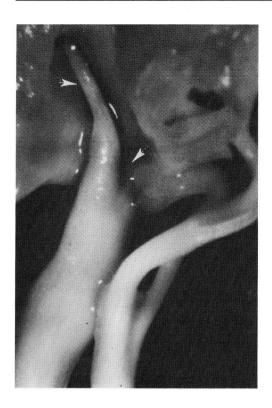

Fig. 6.2. In a sheep the two strands of the same e-PTFE suture fused, having been placed too close on the leaflet side (arrows).

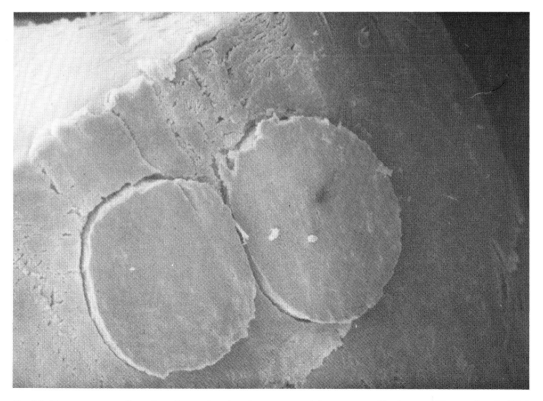

Fig. 6.3. The same case of previous figure showing the two strands incorporated in the same fibrous sheath. SEM.

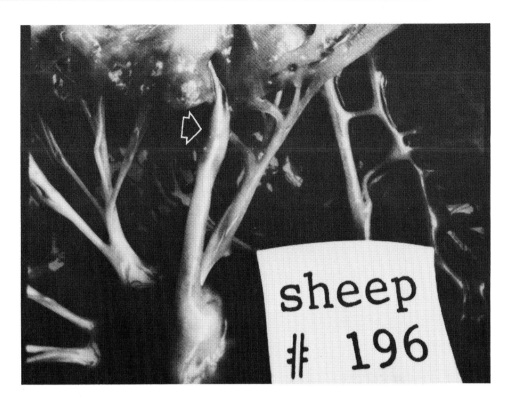

Fig. 6.4. The fusion described in Figs. 6.2 and 6.3 resulted in a neo-chorda (arrow) slightly thicker than natural chordae.

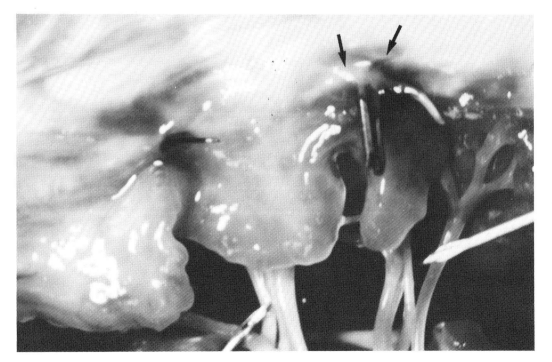

Fig. 6.5. Inflammatory reaction with mild leaflet retraction (arrows) observed in corresponding to a hemoclip utilized to fix artificial chordae in a dog.

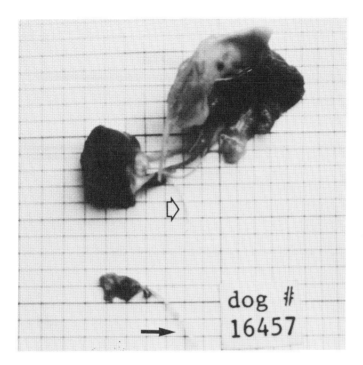

Fig. 6.6. Gravity testing of the degree of bending of artificial chordae (arrow) compared with natural chordae (empty arrow).

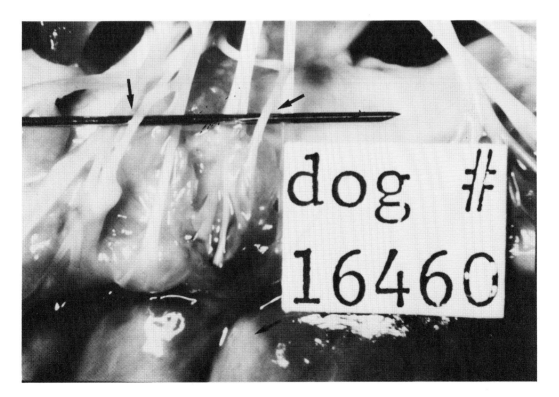

Fig. 6.7. The external appearance and particularly the diameter of artificial chordae (arrows) similar to that of natural chordae after covering by the fibrous sheath.

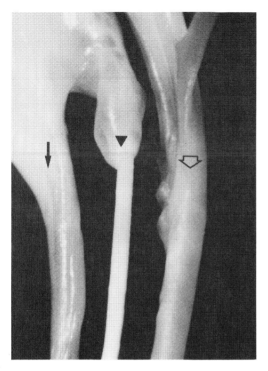

Fig. 6.8. Artificial chorda (arrow) diameter is similar to that of natural chordae (empty arrow) only after fibrous overgrowth, while before it is thinner (triangle).

mens retained their length. Delicate manipulation and bending of leaflets and chordae failed to demonstrate an increased stiffness of artificial structures versus natural ones. The final appearance of Gore-Tex® sutures was absolutely identical to that of the normal natural chordae, so that in some instances only recognition of the small hemoclip on the leaflet side permitted identification of the artificial chordae (Fig. 6.7). As described also by Revuelta,[6] Gore-Tex® sutures seem to provide the skeleton for heart tissues to "generate" new chordae identical in external appearance and function to the natural ones.

MICROSCOPIC EXAMINATION

LIGHT MICROSCOPY

A fibrous sheath covering Gore-Tex® sutures was confirmed with this technique. Only in a few instances was a mild patchy inflammatory infiltrate found (mononuclear cells) at the interface between e-PTFE and fibrous tissue. In one case polymorphonuclear

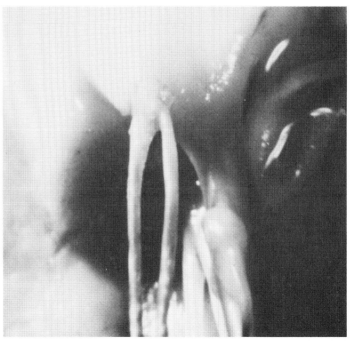

Fig. 6.9. Artificial chordae 13 months after implantation in sheep demonstrate a diameter similar to that found in animals sacrificed after a shorter period after operation.

leukocytes infiltrated the area of insertion of artificial chordae into the leaflet tissue. Transverse sections confirmed mild infiltration of mononuclear cells and neocapillary vessel formation into the fibrous overgrowth near the e-PTFE. The fibrous sheath had a core of dense collagen circumscribed by a thicker layer of less compact fibers with areas of increased cellularity. Finally a thin regular, continuous endothelial layer was present on the surface.

SEM

With this microscopic technique the resemblance of artificial chordae to natural ones was even more evident. The surface of e-PTFE covered by the fibrous sheath appeared smooth, without any thrombi or other blood cell accumulation. It was composed of a monolayer of endothelial cells, strictly oriented along the longitudinal axis of the artificial chordae. Among the areas covered by the fibrous sheath in all specimens, a spot of bare collagen fibers without endothelial cover-

ing was discovered in only one case near the papillary insertion over a pledget (Fig. 6.10). The "columnar" disposition of major connective bundles present in natural chordae was reproduced in artificial ones yielding a structure absolutely indistinguishable—except in cross section—from the former (Fig. 6.11). This confirmed histological observations that e-PTFE sutures constitute the inner portion of the neochorda, represented by the thick compact fibrous core in natural chordae. The surrounding fibrous sheath showed some bridges of collagen fibers infiltrating e-PTFE mostly in the internodal spaces (Fig. 6.12). The areas not yet covered by fibrous overgrowth, in the 6-month specimens, appeared absolutely clean, without any platelet or thrombotic deposition, nor fibroblast colonization. The growing edge of the fibrous sheath was always quite regularly rounded, like a "tissue flow" (Fig. 6.13).

TEM

The fibrous sheath is made by fibroblasts,

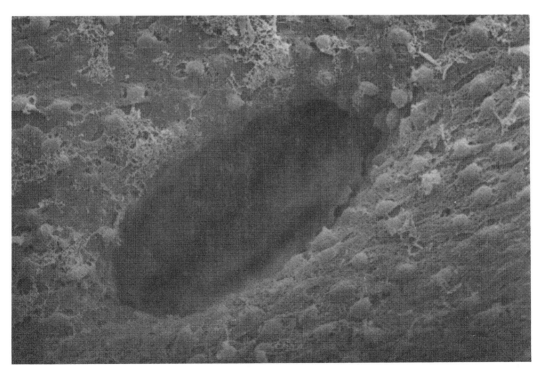

Fig. 6.10. This hole represents the only unexplained area lacking endothelial found among all artificial chordae examined, in correspondence of the insertion on the papillary muscle. SEM.

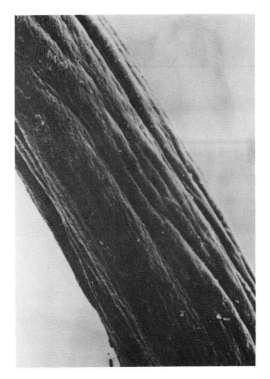
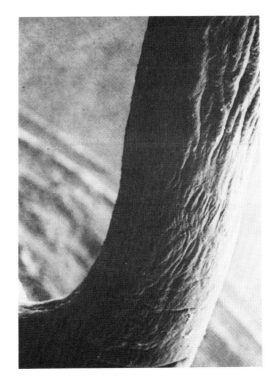

Fig. 6.11 A and B. Regular longitudinal disposition of major connective bundles in natural chordae (A) is reproduced in artificial chordae (B). SEM.

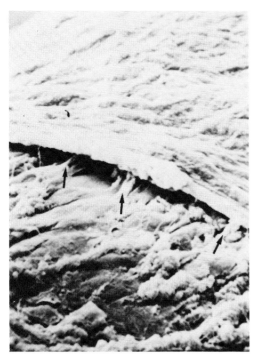

Fig. 6.12. Bridges of fibrous tissue (arrows) infiltrating the internodal spaces of the underlying e-PTFE suture. SEM.

with characteristic elongated nuclei (Fig. 6.14). The disposition of collagen bundles is interesting. Both are oriented longitudinally and radially relative to the major axis of artificial chordae. The external layer of cells was confirmed to be endothelium.

REFERENCES

1. Vetter HO, Burack JH, Factor SM et al. Replacement of chordae tendineae of the mitral valve using the new expanded PTFE suture in sheep. In: Bodnar E, Yacoub M, eds. Biologic and bioprosthetic valves. New York: Yorke Medical Books, 1986:772-84.

2. Frater RWM. Anatomical rules for plastic repair of the diseased mitral valve. Thorax 1964; 19:458-64.

3. Frater RWM, Berghuis J, Brown AL et al. The experimental and clinical use of autogenous pericardium for the replacement and extension of mitral and tricuspid valve cusps and chordae. J Cardiovasc Surg (Torino) 1965; 6:214-28.

4. Frater RWM, Gabbay S, Shore D et al. Reproducible replacement of elongated or

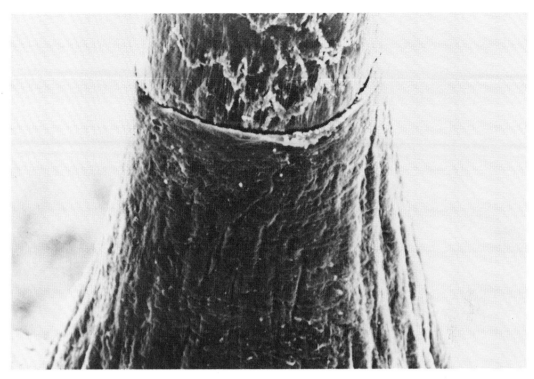

Fig. 6.13. Typical regular rounded edge of fibrous tissue overgrowth. SEM.

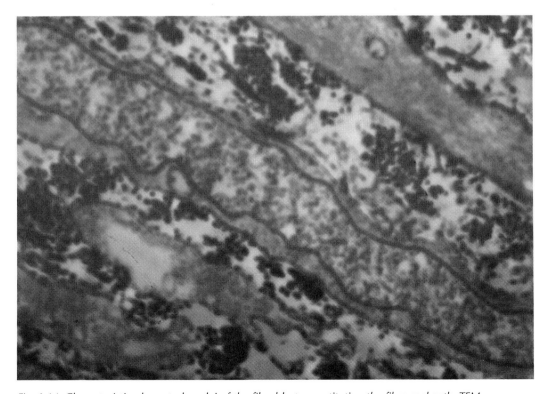

Fig. 6.14. Characteristic elongated nuclei of the fibroblasts constituting the fibrous sheath. TEM.

ruptured mitral valve chordae. Ann Thorac
Surg 1983; 35:14-28.

5. Zussa C, Frater RWM, Galloni SM et al.
Expanded polytetrafluoroethylene as mitral
valve chordae substitute. Proceedings of
Third World Biomaterials Congress. Kyoto,
Japan, April 21-25,1988:128.

6. Revuelta JM, Garcia-Rinaldi R, Gaite L et
al. Generation of chordae tendineae with
polytetrafluoroethylene stents. Results of
mitral valve chordal replacement in sheep.
J Thorac Cardiovasc Surg 1989; 97:98-103.

=CHAPTER 7=

ARTIFICIAL CHORDAE—CLINICAL EXPERIENCE

The final results of the experimental phase of our research became available in October 1986. At that time e-PTFE sutures were not yet approved for clinical cardiac application in the United States. For this reason we started the clinical utilization of artificial chordae in Italy at the Department of Cardiac Surgery of Treviso Regional Hospital, Treviso. We performed the first operation in November 1986. The technique utilized in humans required some minor modifications compared with that in animals. These modifications were produced according to our policy of generating the most "naturally" repaired valve while avoiding any unnecessary artificial material.

First, the use of hemoclips to maintain the length of artificial chordae on the leaflet side was thought unnecessary. Moreover in two animals a mild inflammatory reaction had been observed in the area of contact between hemoclip and leaflet tissue, producing minor retraction, although without any hemodynamic relevance. Therefore in clinical use we tied together the two strands obtained from each suture after connecting each of them with the leaflet.[1] Particular care is paid to maintain at least 2 or 3 mm between the anchoring points of the two arms of the suture to avoid fusion, as observed in one experimental case.

Secondly, since 1989 teflon pledgets, as well as any other artificial material, were not used as prosthetic rings for annuloplasty. Instead autologous pericardium is utilized to create pledgets and reinforcing strips for annuloplasty.

SURGICAL TECHNIQUE

All patients were sedated with oral flunitrazepan (2 mg) and intramuscular fentanyl (1.5 µg/kg) 45 minutes before admission to the operating room. Anesthesia was induced and maintained with fentanyl (50 to 100 µg/kg) and pancuronium (0.2 mg/kg). Sometimes a volatile anesthetic agent (isofluorane) is added at a dosage of 0.4-1%, according to the arterial blood pressure. After orotracheal intubation for mechanical ventilation, the transesophageal echocardiographic probe is inserted and an accurate analysis of all mitral structures is performed with the valve in normal motion.

After opening the chest, pleurae and mediastinal fat are dissected from the anterior surface of pericardium. A rectangular segment (8 x 6 cm) of pericardium is removed and fixed in buffered 0.6% glutaraldehyde (Baxter

Healthcare Corp., Irvine, CA, USA) for 10-15 minutes (Fig. 7.1). After fixation it is rinsed for about 15 minutes in 10 separate saline baths and utilized to manufacture pledgets (Fig. 7.2) and a strip to reinforce suture annuloplasty.

After heparin administration (2-3 mg/kg to maintain the activated coagulation time over 480 seconds), cannulation of the ascending aorta and venae cavae is performed and total cardiopulmonary by-pass is instituted. When mild systemic hypothermia is achieved (28 °C), the aorta is crossclamped and blood-crystalloid (ratio 4:1) cardioplegia is delivered into the aortic root, and repeated every 25-30 minutes throughout aortic cross clamping time.

The left atrium is entered through a standard incision posterior to the right interatrial groove, anterior to the right pulmo-

nary veins.[2] Although this is our access of choice, other accesses were utilized in a few cases, particularly in the presence of a very small left atrium or in reoperation with extensive adhesions. The transseptal approach is one of the more commonly utilized alternatives. Khonsari et al[3] reported a large experience with this access. They enter the right and left atria with a vertical incision that includes the septum from the right superior pulmonary vein to the anterior limbus of the fossa ovalis. A different transseptal approach was utilized by Guiraudon et al.[4]

After entering the right atrium with a longitudinal incision the interatrial septum is incised from the fossa ovalis superiorly to the point where the right atriotomy was carried (between the right atrial appendage and the atrioventricular sulcus). Then, from where the two incisions met, the roof of the left

Fig. 7.1. Autologous pericardium is removed, cleaned from mediastinal fat, fixed for 10 to 15 minutes in buffered 0.6% glutaraldehyde and rinsed ten times.

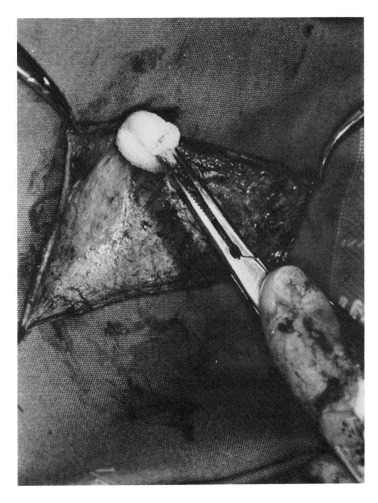

atrium is incised for 3 to 5 cm. A similar approach is utilized by Frater.[5] Both groups reported no early or late complications associated with this technique. Selle[6] and David[4] utilized temporary transection of the superior vena cava to extend the incision in the roof of the left atrium, improving the exposure of the mitral valve. Larbalestier et al[7] dissect the interatrial groove to bring the left atrial incision more anterior and medial; they report superb exposure of the mitral apparatus with any size left atrium, while avoiding injury to the conduction tissue. With any approach a left atrial suction is placed and the atrium is kept widely open with a self-retaining Cosgrove/Kapp atrial retractor (Kapp Surgical Inc., Cleveland, OH, USA).

The mitral valve is carefully examined to verify the correspondence between transesophageal echocardiographic findings and surgical anatomy. Sequential analysis of annular size, leaflet dimension and tissue quality (fibroelastic deficiency or myxomatous degeneration), chordal thinning and elongation (Figs. 7.3 and 7.4) or rupture (Figs. 7.5-7.7) and papillary muscle characteristics is carried out to identify the different procedures requested.

If needed, quadrangular resection is performed first, with two 6-0 Gore-Tex® sutures anchored to the anterior corners of the free edges of the remaining posterior leaflet stumps to retract the cusp, thereby improving papillary muscle exposure (Figs. 7.8-7.11). For the same purpose a sponge is placed under the diaphragmatic surface of the ventricle so that it pushes the posteromedial papillary muscle anteriorly. If posterior chordal rupture is present, the unsupported area is usually included in the resected portion of the leaflet.

When a large resection is required, a sliding maneuver[8] is added to avoid significant plication of the annulus. The leaflet stumps are partially detached from their annular insertion for about 1-1.5 cm each and the posterior corners are then slid to the mid-point of the resection (Figs. 7.12-7.14). The subsequent suture will restore leaflet-annulus continuity gaining progressively on the annular side without any significant plication. When the quadrantectomy must be very large,

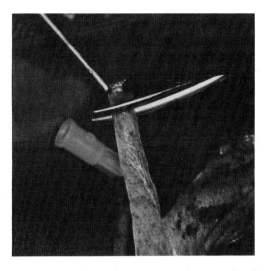

Fig. 7.2. Treated autologous pericardium is utilized to manufacture pledgets and a strip to reinforce annuloplasty.

as in the case of diffuse posterior leaflet chordal elongation and rupture, in order to prevent an insufficient remnant of the posterior leaflet with consequent restrictive valve motion and suture tension, we perform a smaller resection and support instead the residual unsupported areas with artificial chordae.

After quadrangular resection artificial chordae are inserted. Each 5-0 Gore-Tex® suture is anchored to the anterior and posterior components of papillary muscle about 0.5 cm below the tip of the muscle, corresponding to the emergence of ruptured or elongated chordae (Figs. 7.15 and 7.16). The suture is "U" shape. It is reinforced with autologous pericardial pledgets (0.5 x 0.5 cm) on both sides of the muscle and tied very gently to avoid muscle ischemia or tearing (Figs. 7.17-7.19).

As described previously the two strands of the suture are carried, each twice, through the free margin of the unsupported area of the anterior or posterior leaflet (Figs. 7.20-7.22). A small autologous pericardial pledget (0.3 x 0.2 cm) is utilized to reinforce the anchorage on the atrial side of the leaflet (Figs. 7.23 and 7.24).

All needed chordae are placed so as to support the critical areas (Fig. 7.25). Usually when the anterior leaflet is prolapsed all

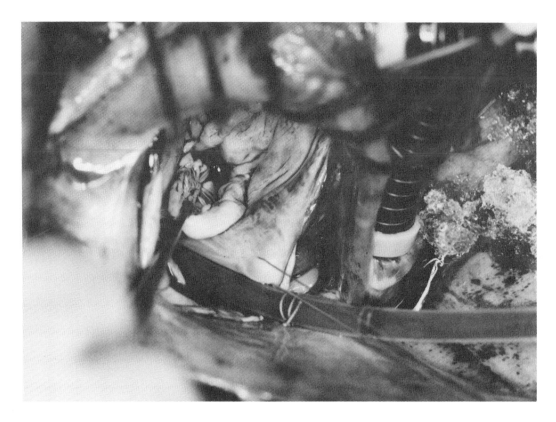

Fig. 7.3. Example of diffuse chordal thinning and elongation.

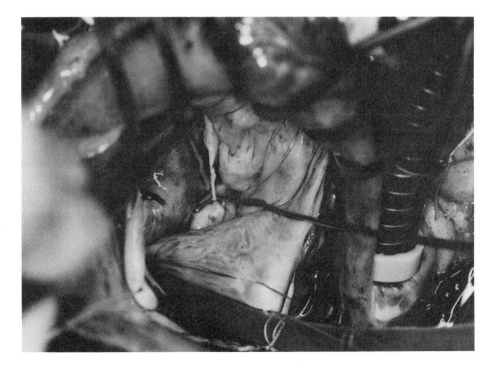

Fig. 7.4. Chordal degeneration with cystic formations in the same patient.

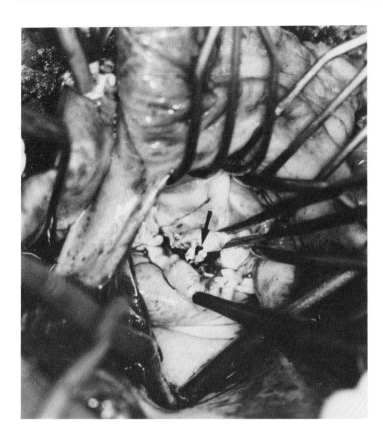

Fig. 7.5. Anterior chordae rupture (arrow) due to endocarditis on a floppy mitral valve.

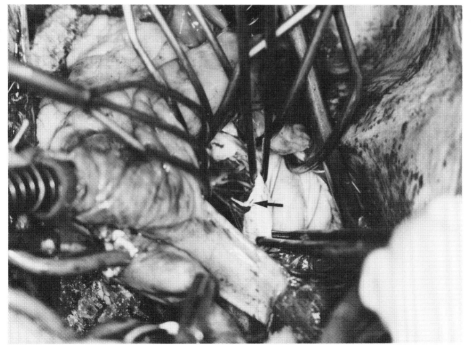

Fig. 7.6. In the same patient as in Figure 5, posterior chordal rupture (arrow) due to the degenerative disease is evident as well.

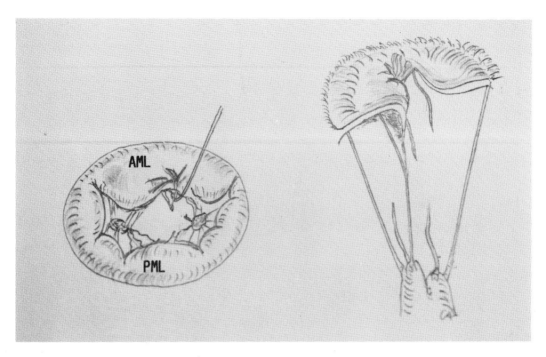

Fig. 7.7. Schematic illustration of the analysis of the valve apparatus to identify all pathological components.

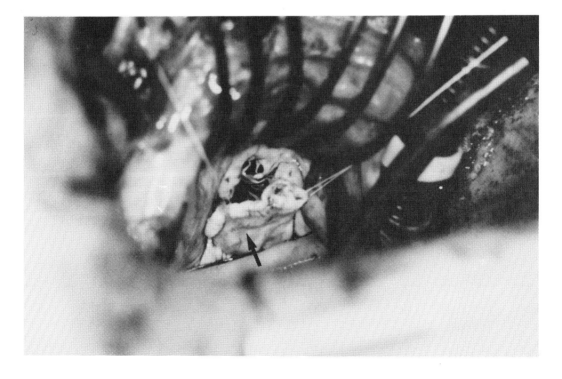

Fig. 7.8. Suspension with two 6-0 Gore-Tex® sutures of the segment of posterior leaflet to be resected (arrow).

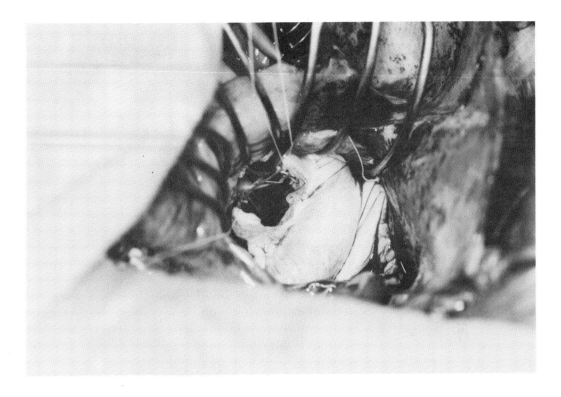

Fig. 7.9. Posterior quadrangular resection performed.

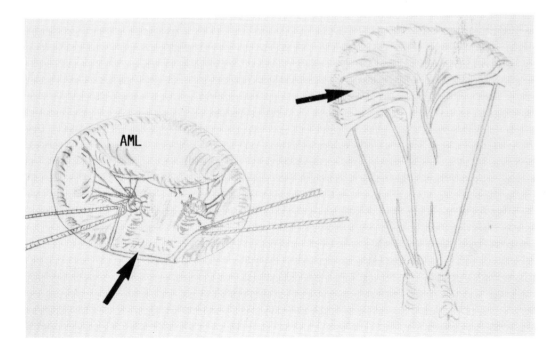

Fig. 7.10. Schematic illustration of the quadrangular resection (arrows).

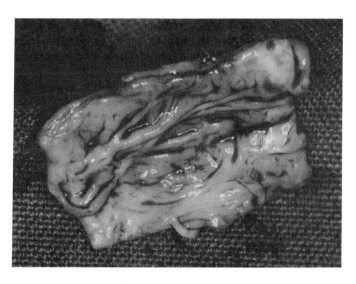

Fig. 7.11. Segment of posterior leaflet resected with anomalous chordal insertions (see Chapter 2, Fig. 2.5).

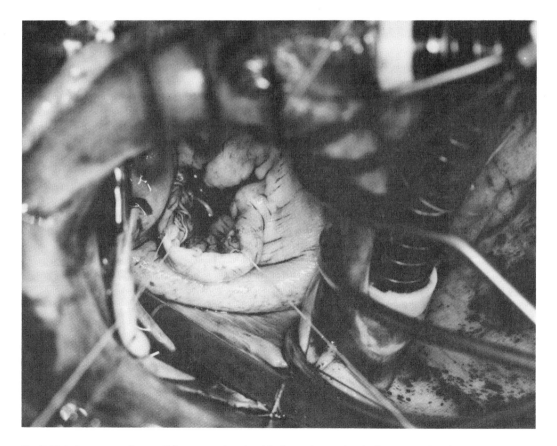

Fig. 7.12. In large resections a sliding procedure is added to reduce subvalvular ventricular plication and suture tension.

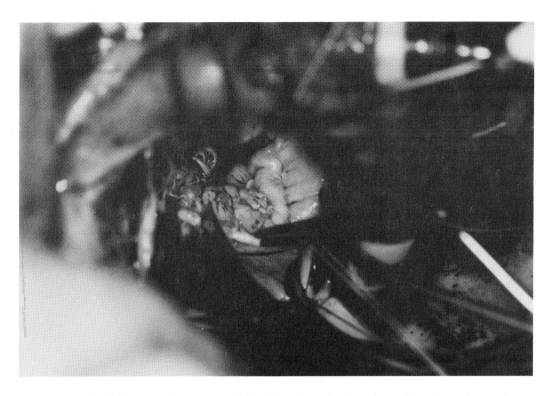

Fig. 7.13. For the sliding procedure two parallel incisions from the free edge to 2 mm from the annulus are made first and the segment of posterior leaflet is removed with an incision connecting the previous two. Continued in the next figure.

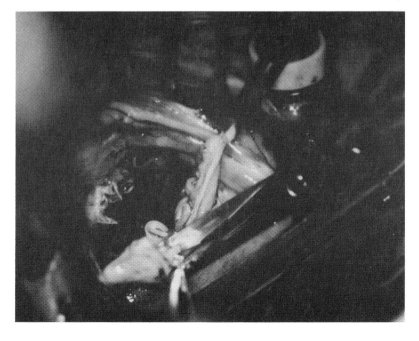

Fig. 7.14. From the corners of the leaflet stumps near the annulus two incisions parallel to the annulus are carried for about 1 to 1.5 cm on each side.

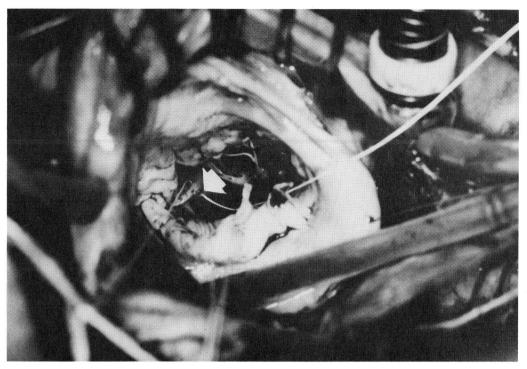

Fig. 7.15. Artificial chorda fixed to the anterior component of the anterolateral papillary muscle (arrow).

along its extension, six sutures are placed, three on each side of the central bare area of the leaflet, obtaining 12 chordae. Almost simultaneously a pair of chordae is placed to stabilize the free margin of the reconstructed posterior quadrantectomy.

The reconstruction of the leaflet is achieved with three or four 6-0 Gore-Tex® sutures. These are applied in an "X" configuration in such a way that the knot is placed on the ventricular surface of the leaflet (Figs. 7.26-7.30). The sliding maneuver is realized with two running 4-0 Gore-Tex® sutures tied together corresponding to the quadrantectomy suture line (Figs. 7.31-7.37).

The annuloplasty is performed (see Chapter 8), sizing the pericardial strip with a Carpentier ring sizer according to the body surface area (BSA) of the patient: size 32 for a BSA below 1.5 m², size 34 for a BSA from 1.5 to 1.8 m², size 36 for a BSA above 1.8 m².

Two different methods of suture are utilized by different surgeons. In one method 8 to 10 interrupted 4-0 Gore-Tex® sutures are anchored to the posterior portion of the annulus, from one fibrous trigone to the other, in a "U" shape and tied after being carried through the inner margin of the pericardial strip, as with the technique used with prosthetic rings (Fig. 7.38). The second method utilizes a 4-0 Gore-Tex® running suture to fix the pericardial strip to the posterior annulus, again from one fibrous trigone to the other. In both cases a 4-0 Gore-Tex® suture is used to fasten the outer margin of the strip to the atrial wall external to the mitral annulus obtaining a smooth surface, avoiding blood flow turbulence (see Chapter 8).

Artificial chordae length is then approximately set pulling the sutures to position the free margins of the leaflets at the same level into the ventricular cavity all along their extension, while maintaining a wide appositional area (Fig. 7.39). The ventricular cavity is then filled with saline solution to close the valve, venting air through an aortic suction. Any residual regurgitant jet is analyzed to correct inadequate apposition. Also the closure line is carefully inspected for symmetry to avoid improper tension. If any further support is thought to be necessary, more artificial chordae are added at this time. Finally, when a satisfactory result is achieved, artificial chordae are tied. This maneuver is crucial to avoid any tension on the sutures to prevent chordal shortening. At the same time square knots are required to prevent release of the sutures.

A final hydrodynamic test with pressure injection of saline solution into the ventricle is performed to assess the result. The left atrium is closed, aortic crossclamp released and cardiopulmonary by-pass discontinued in the standard way. Transesophageal echocardiography is then performed to check the result. Diastolic opening and systolic closure are carefully analyzed to assure satisfactory excursion of the leaflets (Fig. 7.40). In the event echocardiographic findings fail to confirm the positive result observed with the open-heart hydrodynamic test, cardiopulmonary by-pass is reestablished and further procedures—repair or valve replacement—are performed.

A membrane made of PTFE (Gore-Tex® Surgical Membrane) is inserted in all patients to replace the pericardium utilized to reinforce suture annuloplasty and artificial chordae anchorage. This membrane has proved to be very useful in significantly reducing adhesions, facilitating reentry in case of reoperation (Figs. 7.41-7.43).

After almost seven years of clinical experience with artificial chordae insertion, we consider this technique fairly easy. In fact after a short learning period it becomes quite reproducible, keeping in mind a few rules:

(1) The goal of this procedure is to place the corresponding points of the free margins of the leaflets at the same level into the ventricular cavity, obtaining a satisfactory appositional area;

(2) An adequate number of artificial chordae should be utilized in all cases. To support the entire anterior leaflet 8 to 12 chordae (4 to 6 sutures) are usually required, symmetrically distributed on both sides of the bare central area, while four chordae are utilized to support or reduce the posterior

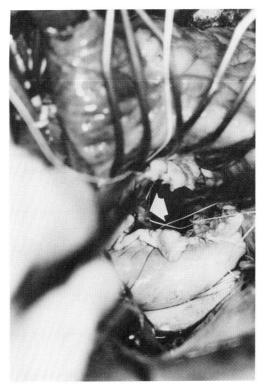

Fig. 7.16. Artificial chorda fixed to the posterior component of the anterolateral papillary muscle (arrow).

quadrangular resection. If commissural chordae were required, two are used for each commissural leaflet;

(3) The final adjustment of artificial chordae length with the valve maintained in closed position, by saline filling of the left ventricular cavity, is mandatory to obtain symmetrical closure and an undistorted appositional area. If there is any doubt that a particular area still lacks adequate support, two more artificial chordae should be inserted at this point. Only after these conditions are satisfied are the artificial chordae tied.

CLINICAL SERIES

From November 1986 to June 1993 110 patients were operated upon utilizing artificial chordae. Demographic data are described in Table 7.1. Ages ranged from 15 to 75 years with a mean of 54 years; the number of males was slightly greater than females (56% versus 43%). More than two-thirds of the patients were in sinus rhythm at the time

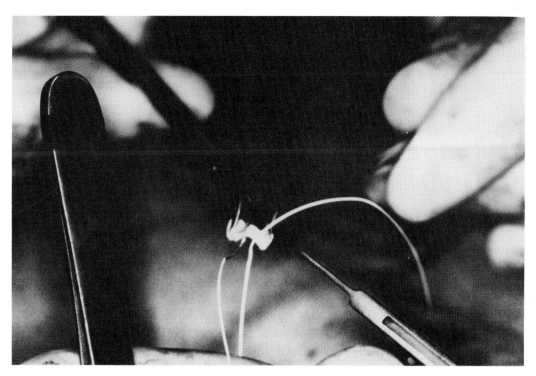

Fig. 7.17. A treated autologous pericardium pledget is utilized to reinforce the anchorage of artificial chordae to the papillary muscle.

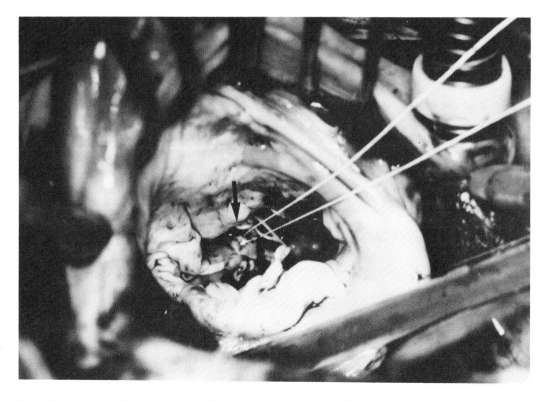

Fig. 7.18. Anterior artificial chordae are then tied very gently to avoid papillary ischemia or tearing.

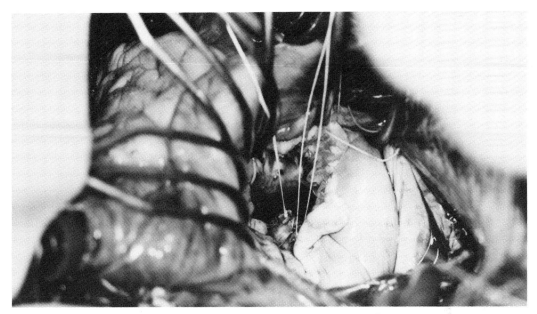

Fig. 7.19. Posterior artificial chordae are tied to the papillary muscle as well.

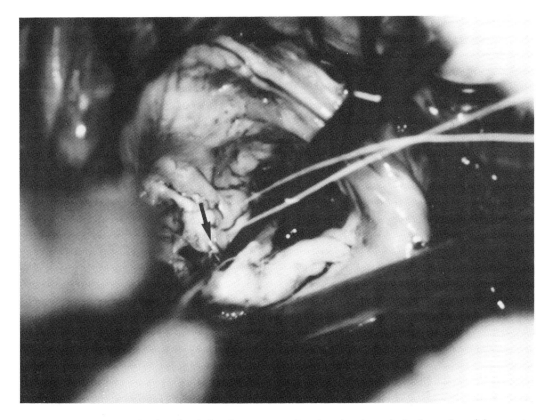

Fig. 7.20. The two strands of artificial chordae are passed each twice through the free edge of the anterior leaflet (arrow) corresponding to the unsupported area.

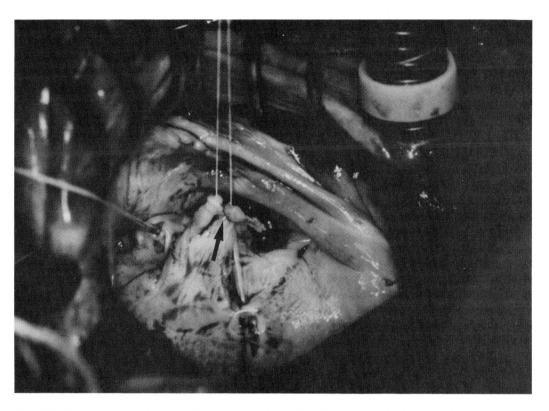

Fig. 7.21. The same procedure (see Fig. 7.20) is performed on the posterior leaflet (arrow).

Fig. 7.22. Schematic illustration of chordal anchorage to the papillary muscle and fixation to the leaflet.

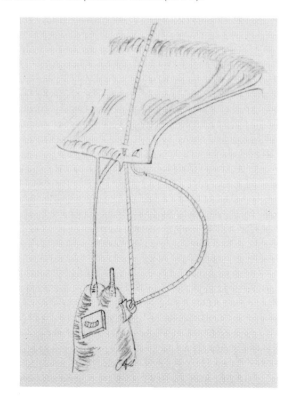

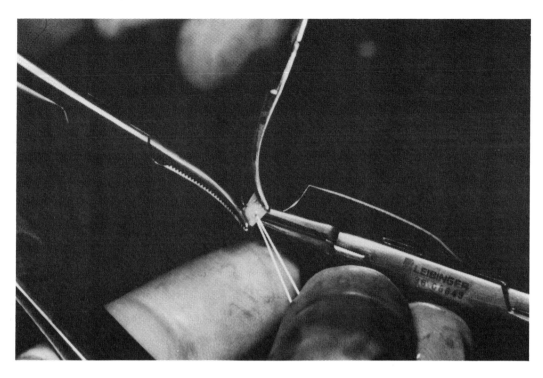

Fig. 7.23. A small treated autologous pericardial pledget is utilized to reinforce artificial chordae fixation to the leaflet.

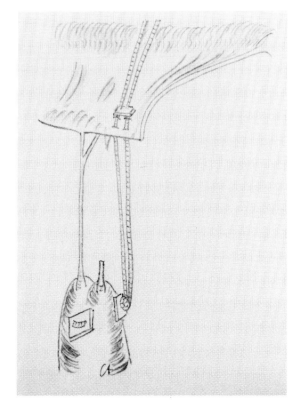

Fig. 7.24. Schematic illustration of the final view of chordal application, before tying.

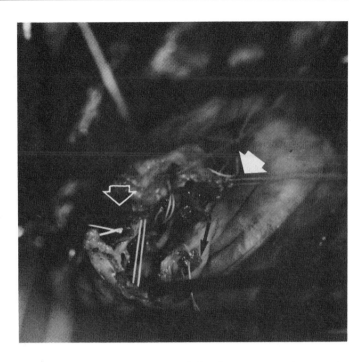

Fig. 7.25. In this phase all required chordae are inserted in anterior (white empty arrow), posterior (black arrow) and commissural position (white arrow).

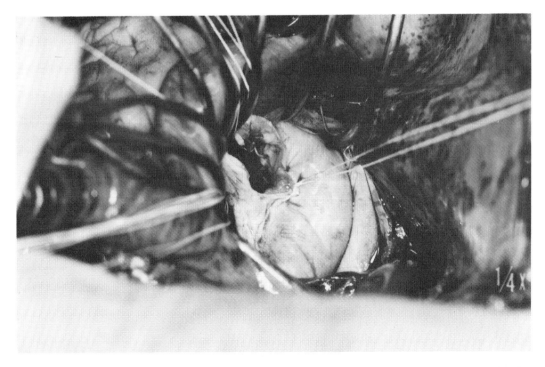

Fig. 7.26. Reconstruction of the quadrangular resection. Usually three 4-0 Gore-Tex® sutures are utilized to close the annular portion of the resection.

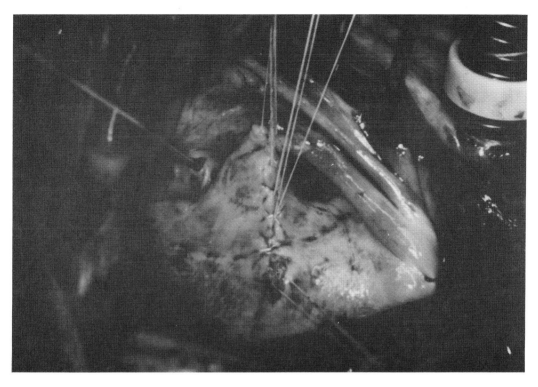

Fig. 7.27. Three or four 6-0 Gore-Tex® sutures are then utilized to close the leaflet portion of the resection. The stitches are passed in "X" shape with the knot on the ventricular surface of the leaflet.

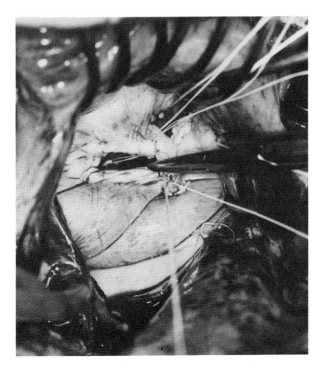

Fig. 7.28. A pair of artificial chordae is usually utilized to support the free edge of the reconstructed resection.

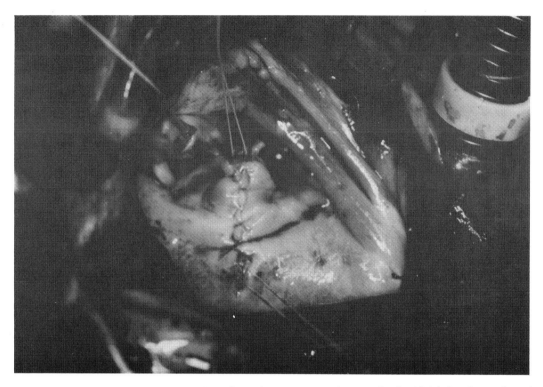

Fig. 7.29. Final view of the reconstructed quadrangular resection with a couple of artificial chordae anchored to the free edge before tying.

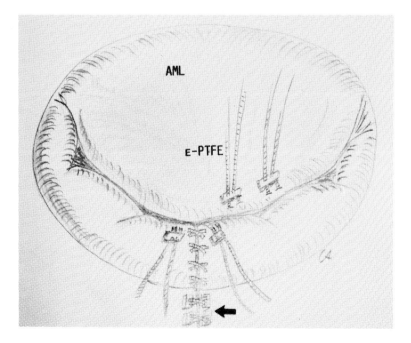

Fig. 7.30. Schematic illustration of reconstructed quadrangular resection (arrow) and artificial chordae fixed to the leaflet, but not tied jet.

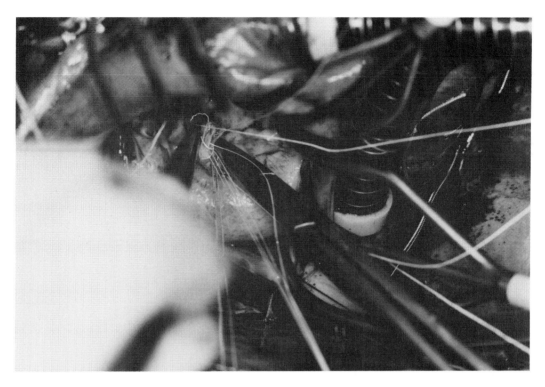

Fig. 7.31. In case of "sliding quadrantectomy," the leaflet portion of the resection is closed in usual way (see Fig. 7.27).

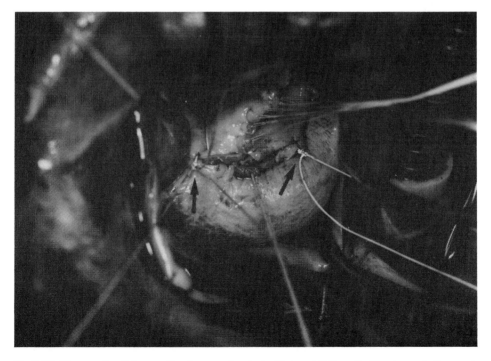

Fig. 7.32. The annular sliding portion is reconstructed with two 4-0 Gore-Tex® sutures starting each from the distal point of the incision (arrows).

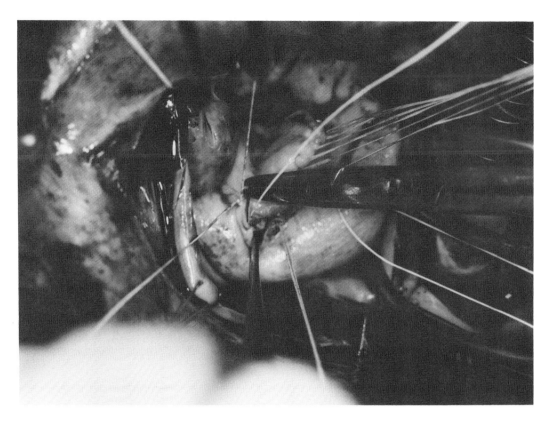

Fig. 7.33. The suture is run to the central point of the quadrantectomy.

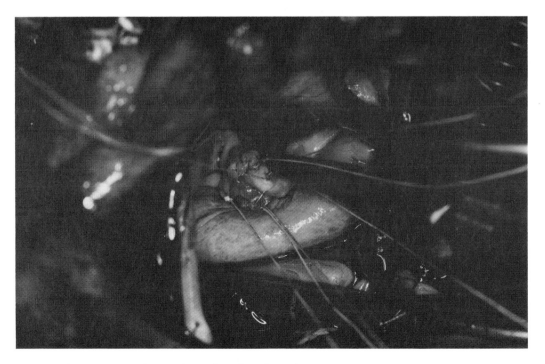

Fig. 7.34. The same procedure performed on the other side.

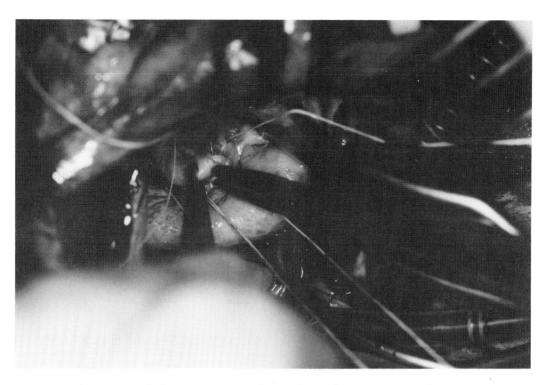

Fig. 7.35. Both sutures reach the point corresponding to the quadrantectomy suture line.

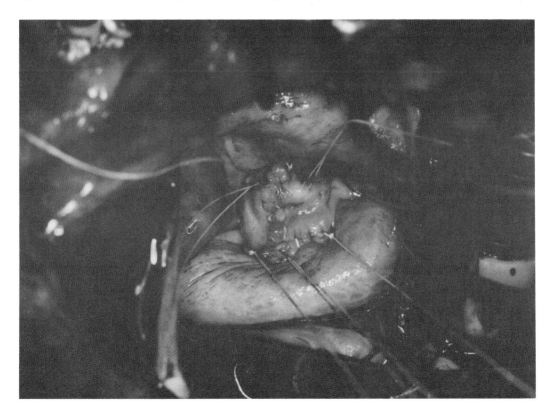

Fig. 7.36. Final view of a reconstructed "sliding quadrantectomy."

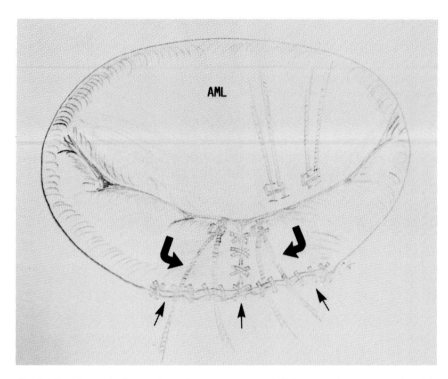

Fig. 7.37. Schematic illustration of a reconstructed sliding quadrantectomy (straight arrows) with the function of this maneuver indicated by curve arrows. AML=anterior mitral leaflet.

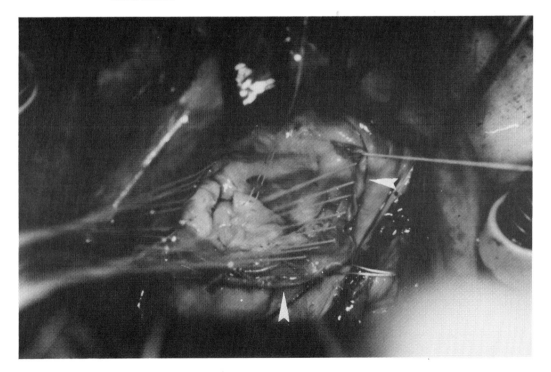

Fig. 7.38. Example of annuloplasty. Eight to ten "U" shaped 4-0 Gore-Tex® stitches are utilized to reduce the length of the posterior annulus, reinforcing with a treated autologous pericardium strip (arrows).

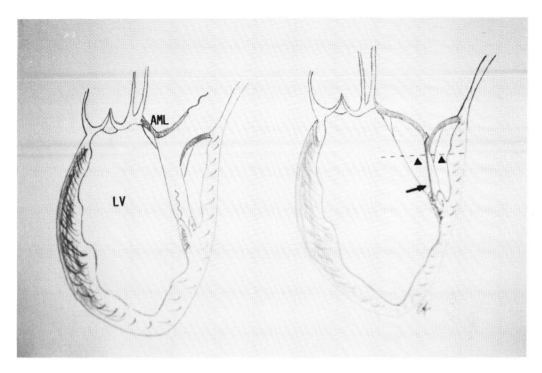

Fig. 7.39. Schematic illustration of the main function of artificial chordae. The free edges of the leaflets are maintained at the same level (triangles) in the ventricular cavity by artificial chordae (arrow), obtaining a wide appositional area. AML=anterior mitral leaflet; LV=left ventricular cavity.

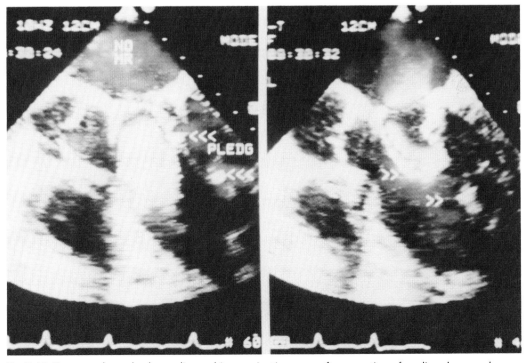

Fig. 7.40. Transesophageal echocardiographic examination soon after cessation of cardiopulmonary by-pass demonstrating absence of mitral regurgitation (NO MR) in systole (left picture) and a wide diastolic valve opening (right picture). Arrows indicate pledgets (PLEDG) utilized to reinforce artificial chordae anchorage.

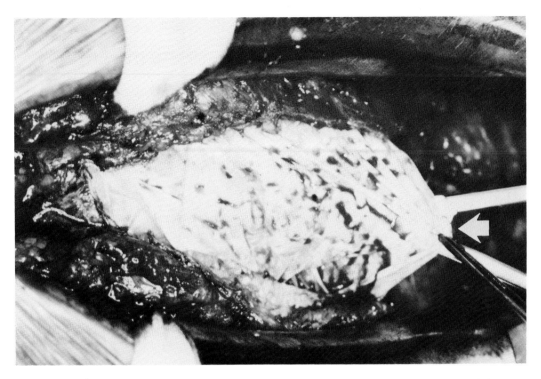

Fig. 7.41. Example of reoperation in a patient with PTFE membrane utilized to close the pericardial cavity at first operation. A surgical instrument is inserted under the membrane (arrow) demonstrating the absence of adhesions.

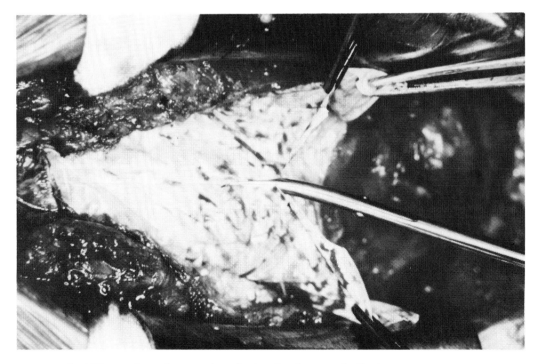

Fig. 7.42. The PTFE membrane is opened confirming the absence of adhesions.

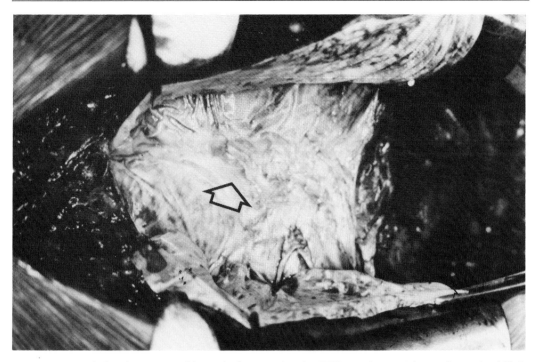

Fig. 7.43. Epicardial surface exposed (arrow) after opening the PTFE membrane. A layer of organized fibrin is present without any adhesion with the surrounding tissues.

of operation; this reflects the increasing number of patients referred before clinical deterioration since reparative procedures havebecome more predictable and reliable. Half of the patients were in functional class III.

The etiology was degenerative in 78% of the patients (floppy mitral valve or fibroelastic deficiency), rheumatic in 17%, and infective or ischemic in the others. The valve was purely insufficient in 87% of the cases and stenotic in 4%; 9% of patients had combined lesions. Concomitant coronary artery disease was noted in 7% of the patients; other valve lesions were present in 8%, an ascending aorta aneurysm in one case and an atrial septal defect in two.

OPERATIVE FINDINGS

The mitral annulus was dilated in most of the cases (85%) and calcified in 4% (Table 7.2). Degeneration (floppy valve or fibro-elastic deficiency) was present in 67 anterior leaflets and 75 posterior leaflets; it was evident in both leaflets in 53 cases (48.2 %). One of these patients had an isolated cleft of the anterior leaflet. This pathology produced prolapse of the anterior leaflet alone in 14

cases, of the posterior in 23 and of both in 63 (57.3%).

Among patients with degenerative pathology chordal alterations (thinning or elongation) were present in more than 90%. Chordal rupture related to the anterior leaflet was detected in 7 cases, to the posterior in 46 and to both in 9. Eighteen of 19 patients with rheumatic disease had fibrotic changes of both leaflets. In 12 of these cases the chordae tendineae and the papillary muscles were involved in the fibrotic process.

CHORDAL SURGICAL PROCEDURE

The number and site of application of artificial chordae is described in Table 7.3. A mean of 6.7 chordae/patient were utilized. In 65% of cases they were inserted in the anterior leaflet position alone or, more commonly, associated with the posterior leaflet position. In 15 cases some supportive chordae were also utilized for commissural tissue. In one case traditional anterior leaflet chordae shortening was associated as well, while in six rheumatic cases chordal splitting was performed.

Table 1. Demographic and clinical data

	n.pts	%
Sex		
Male	62	56.4
Female	48	43.6
Etiology		
Degenerative	86	78.2
Rheumatic	19	17.3
Infective	3	2.7
Ischemic	2	1.8
Valve Lesion		
Insufficiency	96	87.3
Stenosis	4	3.6
Mixed	10	9.1
Rhythm		
Sinus	80	72.7
Atrial Fibrillation	30	27.3
NYHA Functional Class		
I	2	1.8
II	40	36.4
III	55	50.0
IV	13	11.8
Associated Pathologies		
Ischemic	8	7.3
Aortic Valve	4	3.6
Aortic + Tricuspid Valve	5	4.5
Aortic Aneurysm	1	0.9
ASD	2	1.8

	Range	Mean
Age		
Years	15-75	54.2
Pulmonary Wedge Pressure		
"V" Wave	6-65	28.2
Mean	4-38	16.9
Cardiac Index		
l/min/sqm	1.4-5.3	2.8

n. pts=number of patients; NYHA=New York Heart Association; ASD=Atrial Septal Defect; l/min/sqm=liters/minute/square meter of body surface area.

Table 2. Operative findings

	n.pts	%
Valve Annulus		
Normal	12	10.9
Dilated	94	85.5
Calcified	1	0.9
Dilated and Calcified	3	2.7
Anterior Leaflet		
Normal	25	22.7
Degenerated	67	60.9
Fibrotic	18	16.4
Posterior Leaflet		
Normal	10	9.1
Degenerated	79	71.8
Fibrotic	19	17.3
Calcified	2	1.8
Prolapse		
Absent	10	9.1
Anterior	14	12.7
Posterior	23	20.9
Anterior + Posterior	63	57.3
Chordal Rupture		
Absent	48	43.6
Anterior	7	6.4
Posterior	46	41.8
Anterior + Posterior	9	8.2

ASSOCIATED PROCEDURES

In 62 patients quadrangular resection of the posterior leaflet was performed. In three cases calcium debridement and leaflet thinning was carried out, while in one case an isolated cleft of the anterior leaflet was closed. Bilateral commissurotomy was performed in 15 patients. In 103 cases annulolasty was performed: 85 autologous pericardium reinforced suture annuloplasties, 9 simple suture annuloplasties and 9 Carpentier rings. Aortic valve repair was associated in four cases, tricuspid valve repair in three and aortic valve replacement in one. An atrial septal defect was closed in two cases as well.

INTRAOPERATIVE RESULTS

In each case a hydrodynamic test was performed at the end of the procedure by injecting cold saline solution into the left ventricle through the mitral orifice. No regurgitant jets were detected in 76 cases, trivial leakage in 30, a mild jet in 1and significant regurgitation in 3. In these last patients the valve was replaced immediately. They were all operated at the beginning of our experience when the clinical reliability of the technique was still not well-established. The number of chordae inserted in each patient was reduced producing, in some cases, incomplete repair. The positive findings in follow-up enhanced our confidence in this procedure. Accordingly in subsequent operations we placed a greater number of artificial chordae to appose the leaflets, to optimally distribute stress, and to prevent further pathology.

In all patients before September 1988 epicardial echocardiography and thereafter epicardial or transesophageal echocardiography was performed. The patient with a mild regurgitant jet on the hydrodynamic test had moderate mitral insufficiency at transesophageal echocardio-graphy, after weaning from cardiopulmonary by-pass. Therefore mitral valve replacement was performed during the same operation.

EARLY RESULTS

One patient died 15 days after the operation due to respiratory insufficiency. No valve-related complications were reported during the first month after operation.

Transthoracic and transesophageal echocardiography performed before discharge confirmed intraoperative findings. A mean transmitral gradient of 2.1 mmHg (range 0-5) was found, with a mean orifice area of 2.5 sq.cm (range 1.8-3.6). No signs of artificial chordae alterations (detachment, thrombotic deposition, length modifications) could be detected.

Ninety-eight patients were treated for three months with warfarin, unless other conditions like atrial thrombosis or chronic atrial fibrillation with left atrial enlargement required permanent anticoagulation, four with dipyridamole and aspirin and three were discharged without any anticoagulant therapy.

LATE RESULTS

Two patients died two and five months after operation, respectively. The first case was related to renal and respiratory insufficiency and sepsis in a patient that had undergone the operation in cardiogenic shock for papillary muscle rupture after myocardial infarction. The second was due to cardiac insufficiency in a patient with cardiomyopathy and dilatation operated on for triple valve disease.

One patient had a cerebral transient ischemic attack, although treated with warfarin, at the time of sinus rhythm recovery, two months after operation. No other valve-related complications were reported during the follow-up (3 to 82 months, mean 25.3), besides two reoperations described subsequently.

Each patient was followed in the outpatient department with transthoracic echocardiography every six months and transesophageal echocardiography every year. No signs of artificial chordae alterations (thrombi, calcifications, length modifications) have been detected so far. A significant difference has been

Table 3. Artificial chordae. Site of implementation

n.chordae	Anterior		Posterior		Commissural	
	n.pts	%	n.pts	%	n.pts	%
0	38	34.6	30	27.3	94	85.5
2	17	15.5	28	25.5	13	11.8
4	22	20.0	35	31.8	3	2.7
6	14	12.7	13	11.8	-	
8	15	13.6	4	3.6	-	
10	2	1.8	-		-	
12	2	1.8	-		-	

Total Number			Associated Chordal Procedures		
n.chordae	n.pts	%		n.pts	%
2	25	22.7	- Shortening	1	0.9
4	29	26.4	- Splitting	6	5.4
6	13	11.8 8			
8	11	10.0			
10	12	10.9			
12	13	11.8			
>12	7	6.4			

tected so far. A significant difference has been observed however between patients with rheumatic and those with degenerative disease.

Rheumatic patients, in seven cases, had progressive deterioration of valve function with recurrence of regurgitation, although mild in most of the cases. In fact in our preliminary report,[9] among the first 12 patients, 6 had a rheumatic etiology. Except for one patient who underwent mitral valve replacement during the first operation, the other five had a competent valve at six-month follow-up. In later follow-up most had trivial to mild incompetence. So far only one is scheduled for reoperation due to a moderate-severe mitral insufficiency. Our opinion is that this recurrence could be related to the progression of leaflet shrinkage. This opinion is similar to that of other authors.[10-12]

In his large experience with these patients Antunes[10] observed that, although valve repair is performed by a skilled surgeon, late failure is more common than in patients with valve pathology due to a different etiology. This can be explained by the natural evolution of rheumatic pathology, mostly in young people. Lessana and co-workers,[12] analyzing their long-term experience, concluded that while conservative surgery should be applied extensively in patients with degenerative disease, it should be used with caution in cases of rheumatic etiology due to the significantly higher rate of reoperation required in this group of patients.

Our patients with degenerative etiology were stable morphologically and hemodynamically with improved ventricular function. Considering only this group of patients, no significant modifications of valve area and gradient were detected during follow-up.

REOPERATIONS

Two patients required reoperation 18 and 8 months after the first procedure, respectively.

The first patient, operated on at the beginning of our experience, was the only one in whom we combined traditional chordal shortening with artificial chordae insertion. The echocardiographic findings at 6 and 12 months confirmed the absence of any regurgitant jet.

Eighteen months after the surgical procedure sudden mitral regurgitation developed requiring prompt reoperation. Two first order natural chordae of the anterior leaflet, traditionally shortened during the first operation, were broken a few millimeters from the papillary muscle insertion (Fig. 7.44). Also a simple suture annuloplasty was partially dehiscent (Fig. 7.45). The valve was replaced and the patient recovered uneventfully.[13] After this experience we avoided traditional shortening, inserting supportive artificial chordae instead. Also after the introduction of autologous pericardium-reinforced suture annuloplasty we encountered no further suture dehiscence.

In the second case the patient had four artificial chordae inserted posteriorly to replace most of the natural chordae fused and calcified for rheumatic pathology. She was discharged from the hospital with unremarkable echocardiographic findings. Six months later she manifested clinical signs of mitral regurgitation and a transesophageal echocardiography demonstrated a flail posterior leaflet corresponding to the area of insertion of the artificial chordae. At reoperation the one Gore-Tex® suture (two artificial chordae) was untied and the posterior leaflet was consequently flail (Fig. 7.46), although the two strands were still inserted into the free margin of the leaflet. Since the leaflets demonstrated signs of further retraction, the valve was replaced and the patient recovered uneventfully. Since that episode, particular care is taken to make tight square knots, at the same time avoiding excessive tension producing chordal shortening. This was one of the patients in whom a pericardium-reinforced suture annuloplasty was combined with artificial chordae insertion. After eight months the strip of glutaraldehyde treated autologous pericardium was completely covered by endocardium so that it could not be really recognized and consequently explanted. No signs of fibrosis or calcification could be detected and the annulus retained its flexibility. Also the valve orifice diameter was still the size produced by annuloplasty at first operation.

In both cases we could not find any thromboti or calcification of artificial chordae, macroscopically. Length was retained, and healing to papillary muscles and leaflet tissue was perfect.

As previously demonstrated in animal experiments, light and scanning electron microscopy confirmed that Gore-Tex® chordae were partially (1 to 1.5 cm of length) covered by a fibrous sheath growing from papillary and leaflet sides (Fig. 7.47-7.49). The longitudinal disposition of major connective bundles, as observed in natural chordae, was confirmed as well (Fig. 7.50 and 7.51). The surface of the fibrous sheath was absolutely smooth, with a regular array of endothelial cells (Fig. 7.52-7.54). The portion of suture still uncovered was free of thrombi (Fig. 7.55 and 7.56). Microscopy confirms that e-PTFE sutures comprise the thick, inner, compact fibrous core present in natural chordae (Fig. 7.57-7.60).

INDICATIONS FOR ARTIFICIAL CHORDAE INSERTION

Based on our 80-month experience with e-PTFE chordae insertion the indications for this procedure have changed during recent years. In fact they are now more extensive in cases of degenerative pathology and more restrictive for rheumatic etiology.

As we became more confident in the procedure and were encouraged by the results of medium-term follow-up, we opted to utilize artificial chordae more liberally. We insert e-PTFE chordae to support areas with pathological chordae, i.e., elongated and thinned, even if valve incompetence is not actually present in that area. This is intended to avoid recurrence of mitral regurgitation due to further chordal dysfunction.

In rheumatic disease we are more restrictive in our use of artificial chordae since our experience suggested that the final fate of rheumatic valves is dependent more on progression of leaflet scarring than on elongation of affected chordae. We utilize artificial chordae in these cases only if leaflet tissue is still in satisfactory condition without reduced

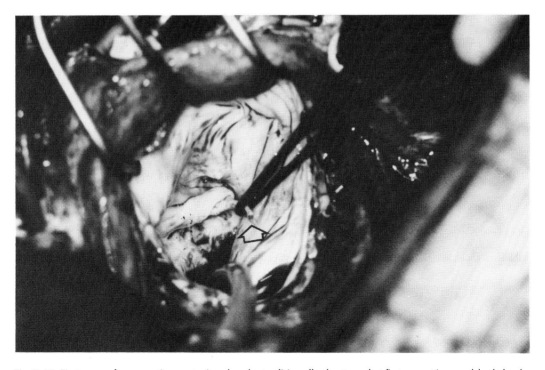

Fig. 7.44. First case of reoperation: anterior chorda, traditionally shortened at first operation, suddenly broke 18 months later (arrow).

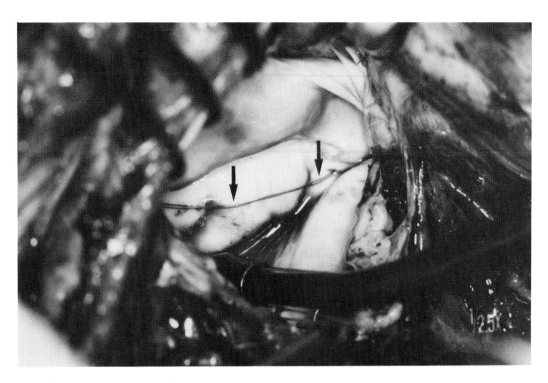

Fig. 7.45. In the same patient of Figure 44, dehiscence of a simple suture annuloplasty (arrows) was found as well.

Fig. 7.46. Second case of reoperation: the knot of one pair of artificial chordae (empty arrows) were found released (arrows) due to a technical error producing a flail posterior leaflet.

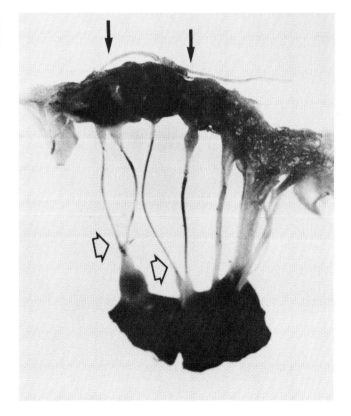

pliability and chordae are affected only in isolated areas.

Our current indications to insert artificial chordae are:

(1) Anterior ruptured chordae associated with posterior prolapsed or flail cusp;

(2) Elongated chordae that are excessively thin and arise from a broad extent of papillary muscles, or from very thin or sessile papillary muscles, as in case of fibroelastic deficiency;

(3) Flail posterior leaflet too severe to be corrected only with a large quadrangular resection;

(4) Supportive, in cases of diffuse degeneration, also to areas not actually insufficient;

(5) Isolated thick or calcified anterior chordae; and

(6) cCmmissural prolapse produced by extensive commissurotomy associated with poor support of the commissural tissue.

In our patient population the last two indications are now diminishing and cases of rheumatic valve disease are ever more rare.

REFERENCES

1. Zussa C, Valfre' C, Frater RWM et al. Artificial chordae in the treatment of mitral valve pathology. In: Ghosh PK, Unger F, eds. Cardiac Reconstructions. Berlin: Springer-Verlag, 1989:207-10.
2. Balasundaram SG, Duran C. Surgical approaches to the mitral valve. J Cardiac Surg 1990; 5:163-9.
3. Khonsari S, Sintek CF. Transatrial approach revisited. Ann Thorac Surg 1990; 50:1002-3.
4. David T. Discussion of: Guiraudon GM, Ofiesh JG, Kaushik R: Extended vertical transatrial septal approach to the mitral valve. Ann Thorac Surg 1991; 52:1058-62.
5. Frater RWM. Discussion of: Guiraudon GM, Ofiesh JG, Kaushik R: Extended vertical transatrial septal approach to the mitral valve. Ann Thorac Surg 1991; 52:1058-62.
6. Selle JC. Temporary division of the superior vena cava for exceptional mitral valve

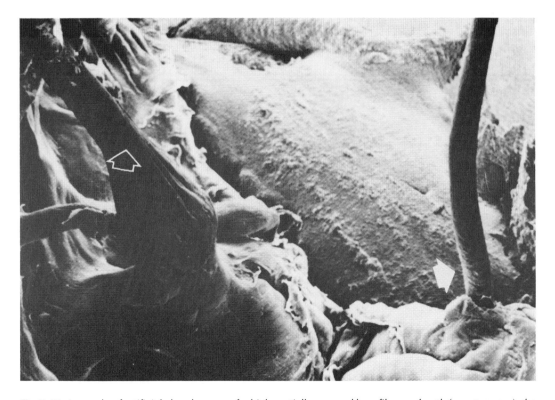

Fig. 7.47. A couple of artificial chordae one of which partially covered by a fibrous sheath (empty arrow), the other still completely uncovered (arrow), eight months after implantation. SEM.

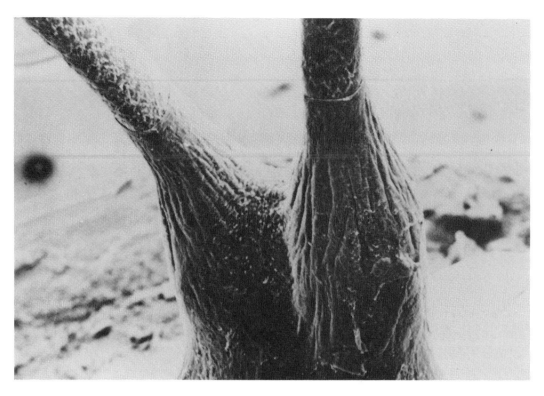

Fig. 7.48. Both strands of a couple of artificial chordae are partially covered by fibrous overgrowth from the papillary muscle, 18 months after implantation. SEM.

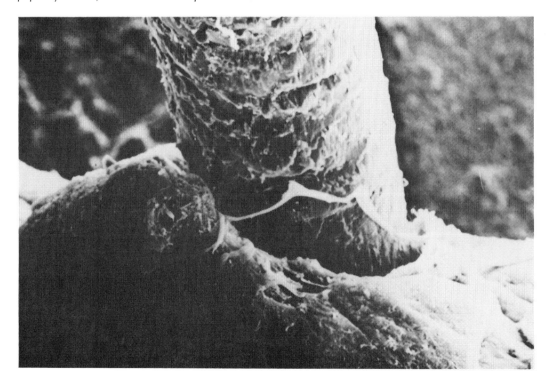

Fig. 7.49. One artificial chorda completely uncovered eight months after implantation. SEM.

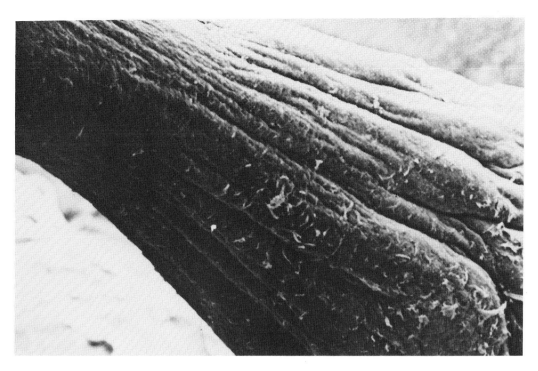

Fig. 7.50. Artificial chorda showing longitudinal disposition of major connective bundles as observed in natural chordae. SEM.

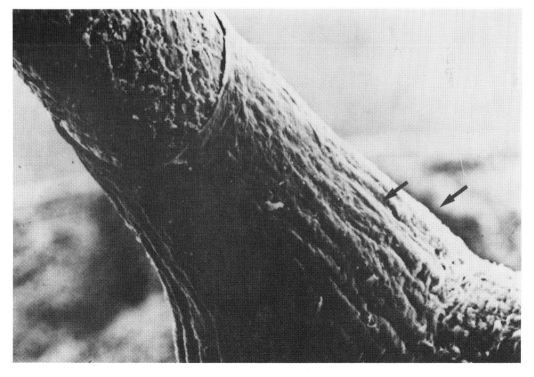

Fig. 7.51. The proximal portion of the fibrous sheath demonstrates the longitudinal disposition of connective bundles (arrows), while the distal portion is still very thin and not completely organized. SEM.

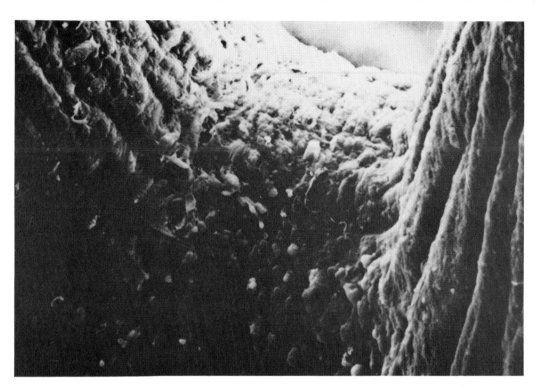

Fig. 7.52. Endothelial cells array at bifurcation of a pair of artificial chordae on the papillary side. SEM.

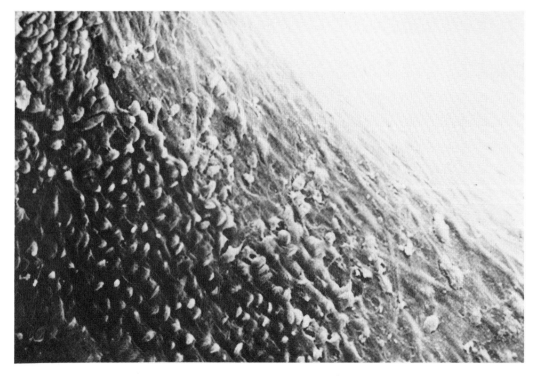

Fig. 7.53. Area of endothelial growth. The surfaces of the endothelized and non-endothelized areas are smooth without any thrombi. SEM.

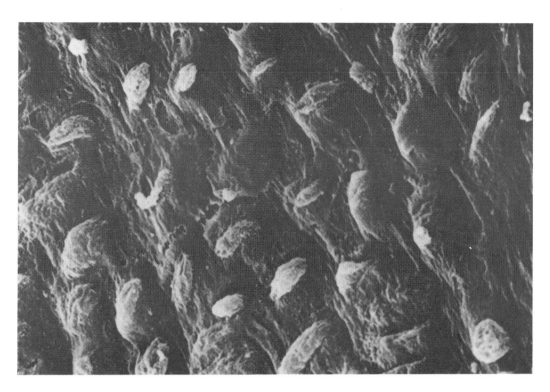

Fig. 7.54. At higher magnification the regular array of endothelial cells covering the fibrous sheath over artificial chordae is demonstrated. SEM.

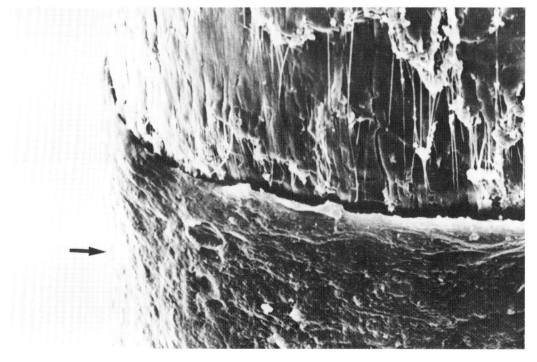

Fig. 7.55. Line of tissue overgrowth showing a regular edge and absence of thrombi over the fibrous sheath (arrow). SEM.

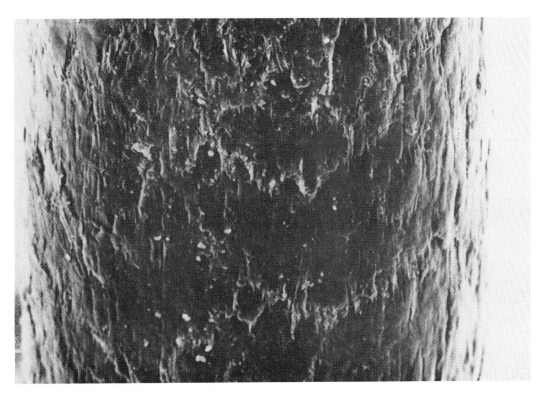

Fig. 7.56. Same chorda of the previous figure showing a clean surface also in the still uncovered portion of e-PTFE. SEM.

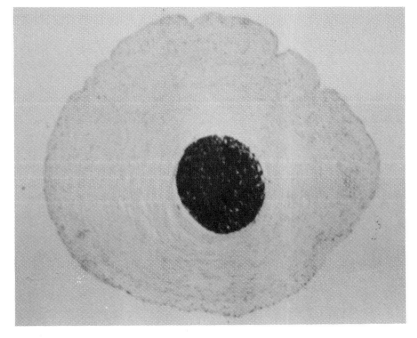

Fig. 7.57. Transverse section of artificial chorda 18 months after implantation showing the core represented by e-PTFE suture, the fibrous sheath and the surrounding endothelial layer. H-E stain.

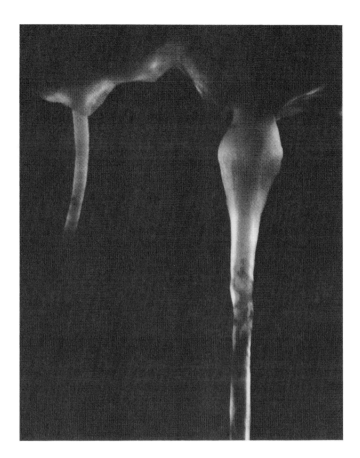

Fig. 7.58. With polarized light the function of the skeleton represented by e-PTFE suture is evident in partially covered neo-chorda (right), while on the left side the suture is still uncovered.

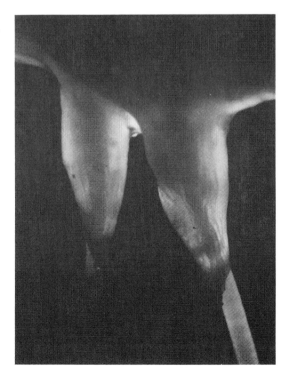

Fig. 7.59. In this example both strands of the same suture show the function of the inner core in neo-chordae formation. Polarized light.

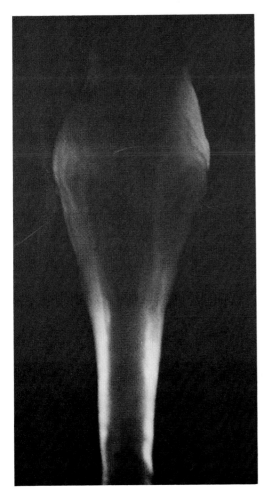

Fig. 7.60. At higher magnification the inner core represented by e-PTFE suture and the surrounding fibrous overgrowth is clearly demonstrated. Polarized light.

exposure. J Thorac Cardiovasc Surg 1984; 88:302-4.

7. Larbalestier RI, Chard RB, Cohn LH. Optimal approach to the mitral valve: Dissection of the interatrial groove. Ann Thorac Surg 1992; 54:1186-8.

8. Deloche A, Jebara VA, Relland JYM et al. Valve repair with Carpentier techniques. The second decade. J Thorac Cardiovasc Surg 1990; 99:990-1002.

9. Zussa C, Frater RWM, Polesel E et al. Artificial mitral valve chordae: Experimental and clinical experience. Ann Thorac Surg 1990; 50:367-73.

10. Antunes MJ. Mitral valvuloplasty for rheumatic heart disease. Semin Thorac Cardiovasc Surg 1989; 1:164-75.

11. Loop FD. Long-term results of mitral valve repair. Semin Thorac Cardiovasc Surg 1989; 1:203-10.

12. Lessana A, Carbone C, Romano M et al. Mitral valve repair: Results and decision-making process in reconstruction. Report of 275 cases. J Thorac Cardiovasc Surg 1990; 99:622-30.

13. Zussa C, Frater RWM, Polesel E et al. Artificial mitral valve chordae: Clinical experience. In: Bodnar E, ed. Surgery for heart valve disease. London: ICR Publishers, 1990:375-82.

=CHAPTER 8=

ANNULOPLASTY

Since annuloplasty is a crucial component of almost any reparative procedure on insufficient mitral valves, I will discuss the function of and various methods available for this procedure.

ANNULAR SHAPE AND FUNCTION

Starting from the distinctions in leaflet-annular relationships frequently observed in intersecting echocardiographic views, in 1987 Levine et al[1] constructed a model to analyze the variations of mitral annulus geometry throughout the cardiac cycle. Echocardiographic observations assume the mitral annulus is in a Euclidean plane. Mitral prolapse is defined when leaflet displacement above this plane is observed during systole. According to this criterion in some cases this phenomenon is evident in one view, i.e., apical four-chamber view, yet is absent in the orthogonal parasternal long-axis view. Therefore Levine tested a different hypothesis: that the plane of the mitral annulus has a saddle shape, with the highest points located anteriorly and posteriorly, while the leaflets have a surface concave toward the ventricular cavity due to the closing pressure counterbalanced by chordal tension. Testing this hypothesis in vitro and in a series of clinically normal individuals, the authors confirmed their assumption of a nonplanar systolic configuration of the annulus that explains the discrepancy between observations in orthogonal echocardiographic views. Indeed in a four-chamber view the leaflets appear to be displaced above the annular plane, while actually they don't reach the highest points of this plane that are examined with the parasternal long-axis view.

The sphincter-like function of the mitral annulus was described by Davis and Kinmonth in 1963.[2] In systole annular contraction reduces the valve area by about 26%. Also the shape of the annulus changes throughout the cardiac cycle, being circular in diastole and elliptical in systole. These modifications of annular shape are determined by contraction and relaxation of basoconstrictor muscles which also play a role in the sequential contraction of the left ventricular basal area.[3,4] Ormiston et al[5] confirmed the 26% reduction of systolic annular area as well as the variations of shape throughout cardiac cycle. van Rijk-Zwikker et al[6] also demonstrated in experimental models that the mitral annular dimension is influenced by the interplay of contraction and dilatation of the left atrium and ventricle as well as by changes in load and in inotropy. Similar findings have been described by Handschumacher et al[7] in a dynamic three-dimensional reconstruction of the normal mitral valve obtained by echocardiography.

All of these observations[1-2] raise the question whether traditional techniques for mitral annuloplasty interfere with these physiologically important functional changes of the mitral annulus.

ANNULOPLASTY

Several annuloplasty techniques have been proposed by different authors. Wooler,[8] Kay[9] and Reed[10] utilized similar methods to plicate the annulus at the commisural areas, reducing the extension of the posterior annulus. A different approach was proposed by Paneth et al.[11] They utilized the so called "mitral plication suture" that employs a double-armed suture, reinforced with a Teflon pledget, placed at the margin of the central fibrous body and runs around the annulus to the posterior portion where it is tied over a second pledget. A second suture is correspondingly placed on the opposite side, if necessary, starting from the other fibrous trigone. The rationale for this technique is reduction of the size of the mitral annulus and at the same time correction of regurgitation confined to one-half of the valve.

Carpentier[12] examined the characteristic features of annular dilatation and proposed the application of a rigid prosthetic ring. He observed that dilatation is confined to the mural leaflet and commissural areas, while the anterior portion between fibrous trigones is never affected. Also dilatation is an ongoing process that produces a deformation of the annular shape so that the anteroposterior diameter is greater than the transverse diameter. Consequently he suggested the use of a semi-rigid ring that could restore valve area as well as annular shape, stabilizing this structure in a systolic position. The ring is pre-shaped and pre-sized to fit the surface area of the anterior leaflet.

Duran[13-14] proposed a flexible ring that could conform to changes in shape of the mitral annulus throughout the cardiac cycle. The theoretical advantage of this kind of flexible ring is that it avoids the possible diastolic stenosis produced by the rigid ring that fixes the valve in the systolic shape and area. Another flexible ring was proposed by Puig Massana.[15] This device has the added feature of being adjustable in size after implantation. Other rings are becoming available as well. All of these new devices are, at least partially, flexible and, in most cases, adjustable in size and shape, even asymmetrically.[16]

COMPARISON BETWEEN DIFFERENT PROCEDURES

All attempts to improve ring characteristics are suggested by the results of comparative experimental and clinical studies of various annuloplasty techniques. As emphasized by Duran,[17] the ideal annuloplasty is physiologically flexible varies in size and shape in diastole and systole.

David[18-19] examined the impact of rigid versus flexible rings on left ventricular function in two groups of patients with chronic mitral regurgitation. Postoperative end-diastolic diameter and volume decreased in both groups. Systolic function, expressed as end-systolic diameter and volume as well as pressure-volume relationship and stroke volume—end-diastolic volume relationship, was significantly better in patients with flexible ring. These data were confirmed up to three months after operation. In a small subgroup of patients studied one year later, no significant differences could be demonstrated.[19] This suggests that the left ventricle continues to improve for a long period after operation and that this improvement produces compensatory mechanisms that reduce the negative effect of fixation of the mitral annulus.

These findings may partially explain conclusions obtained in an experimental model by Rayhill et al.[20] They found that rigid fixation of the mitral annulus doesn't influence global and regional left ventricular function. These data were obtained in open-chest dogs with normal heart before operation. The same authors stated that the effects of rigid fixation of the mitral annulus may not be transposed to chronically diseased left ventricles, as in long-standing mitral regurgitation. Indeed the positive effect of flexible annuloplasty is appreciable early after operation when compared with rigid annuloplasty, while it is not detectable later when left ventricular functional improves significantly.[19]

Comparing suture annuloplasty with mitral valve replacement in chronic mitral regurgitation, Sakai et al[21] confirmed the beneficial effect of the former on ventricular systolic performance. This was related by the authors to the preservation of annular contraction and ventriculo-annular continuity.

On the other hand, in cases of ischemic mitral regurgitation, Czer et al[22] compared ring versus suture annuloplasty. They found similar one-year survival and NYHA functional class in both groups, while ring annuloplasty resulted in lower residual regurgitation and a larger success rate (more than a two grade of mitral regurgitation reduction), probably due to greater reduction of annular diameter and more uniform shortening of the annulus. This second element is explained by the type of suture annuloplasty utilized, the Kay commissural annuloplasty.[9] However a rigid ring produces a smaller valve area and a higher mean gradient.

In a recent paper van Rijk-Zwikker et al[6] examined the effects of rigid versus flexible rings utilizing cinefluoroscopy and videoendoscopy. They found that flexible rings interfere less with the movements of the annulus and the basal part of the left ventricle, although the differences for physiological pressure values were not significant. Also rigid rings may cause mild subaortic obstruction by pushing the annulus anteriorly during systole. This phenomenon was studied by Lee et al.[23] They reported a 2.5% incidence of left ventricular outflow tract obstruction associated with a large redundant posterior leaflet, nondilated left ventricular cavity and consequent anterior displacement of the coaptation line, after mitral valve repair. Jebara and co-workers[24] reported 14% incidence of this complication after prosthetic ring insertion in the high risk group of patients with the previously described anatomical characteristics. Since 1988 they have utilized the sliding technique proposed by Carpentier[25] obtaining a significant reduction of incidence and severity of subvalvular gradients. This maneuver reduces the height of the posterior leaflet and avoids excessive plication of the posterior annulus reconstructing quadrangular resections.

Another complication associated with the utilization of prosthetic rings or other artificial materials for mitral valve repair is hemolysis. Two recent reports by Wilson et al[26] and Dilip et al[27] described severe hemolysis requiring reoperation after mitral valve repair. In the first paper the authors[26] reported two cases of this complication related to a residual regurgitant jet hitting a Duran ring utilized for annuloplasty. Dilip[27] described a similar event due to a jet directed against teflon pledgets used to repair a quadrangular resection. Also David et al[28] reported one instance of severe hemolysis in a case in which a ring annuloplasty was combined with artificial chordae implantation. A trivial regurgitant jet was directed against the artificial ring that was found uncovered by endocardium in that area at reoperation nine months after the first procedure.

Therefore the best procedure for mitral annuloplasty is still controversial and further research is needed to resolve problems and obtain a satisfactory functional result.

PERICARDIUM REINFORCED SUTURE ANNULOPLASTY

Our experience in mitral annuloplasty may be divided into three phases. In the first period (1985-87) our procedure of choice was suture annuloplasty modified from that proposed by Paneth and co-workers.[11] Both arms of a double-armed 3-0 polypropylene suture were run from one fibrous trigone to the other along the posterior annulus reinforcing it with teflon pledgets at both end points. The suture was pulled to reduce the annular size to a predetermined diameter calibrated with an obturator of our design. In the same period a few Carpentier rings were utilized in particular cases when dilatation was associated with severe deformation of the annulus. During the follow-up of patients treated with the suture annuloplasty (66 cases), we observed seven instances of suture dehiscence producing mitral regurgitation requiring reoperation. For this reason we started a second phase, lasting about one year, in which we expanded the indications for the Carpentier ring (23 cases).

We didn't observe any of the complications described with this device and no patient has required reoperation for any cause so far. Yet despite the satisfactory results obtained with the Carpentier ring, our efforts to avoid the disadvantages described by other authors when a rigid ring is utilized and our policy to reduce as much as possible the implantation of artificial materials in mitral position encouraged us to seek a new procedure that could also prevent the complications observed with simple suture annuloplasty. Some authors proposed the use of pericardium to reconstruct the mitral annulus or to reinforce the annuloplasty. David[29] successfully utilized this material to reconstruct the mitral annulus in cases of infective or iatrogenic disruption. Salati[30] and Hendren[31] use pericardium to reinforce suture annuloplasties. When we introduced autologous pericardial pledgets in artificial chordae implantation in 1989, we began using the same material for annuloplasty (third phase).[32]

SURGICAL TECHNIQUE

A rectangular patch of autologous pericardium is fixed in buffered 0.6% glutaraldehyde (Baxter Healthcare Corp., Irvine, CA, USA) for 10-15 minutes. It is then rinsed in saline solution following the same procedure utilized with bioprostheses. In accordance with the body surface area (BSA) of the patient, a strip of pericardium is tailored to reproduce the posterior annulus utilizing a Carpentier ring sizer. For a BSA below 1.5 m^2 a sizer 32 is used, for a BSA from 1.5 to 1.8 m^2 a sizer 34 and a sizer 36 if BSA is above 1.8 m^2 (Figs. 8.1-8.3).

The inner margin of the strip (toward the leaflet) is anchored to the posterior mitral annulus from one fibrous trigone to the other with eight to ten interrupted "U" shaped 4-0 Gore-Tex® sutures (Figs. 8.4-8.10) or, alternatively, with two running 4-0 Gore-Tex® sutures each starting from one trigone (Figs. 8.11-8.14). To correctly identify the site of fibrous trigones we perform the maneuver suggested by Duran (personal communication). Pulling on the central area of the free margin of the anterior leaflet, two wrinkles are produced on the surface on the leaflet. Their directions toward anterior mitral annulus indi-

cate the sites of the fibrous trigones (Fig. 8.15). With both techniques the outer margin of the strip is then fixed to the atrial wall with a running 4-0 Gore-Tex® suture (Figs. 8.16-8.20) to obtain a smooth surface, to avoid flow turbulence, and to better distribute the stress on the annuloplasty involving the atrial wall.

CLINICAL SERIES

So far 94 patients have been operated upon utilizing a pericardium-reinforced suture annuloplasty. One patient died 15 days after operation because of respiratory failure, while three patients died during follow-up. None of these late deaths were related to the mitral procedure; they were due to an associated ischemic cardiac disease.

Three other patients have been reoperated upon so far, 18, 13 and 7 months after the first procedure. The causes of reoperation were failure of aortic valve reconstruction in one case, recurrence of a ventricular aneurysm in another and a technical error in tying artificial chordae in the last. In all three cases the pericardial strip utilized for annuloplasty was completely covered by endothelium, and it was also impossible to recognize the sutures utilized to anchor the strip. The annulus was completely flexible without any detectable sign of fibrosis or calcification. The diameter of the mitral orifice had retained the size produced with the annuloplasty at first operation.

No cases of recurrent mitral regurgitation, hemolysis or anterior displacement of the leaflets, producing outflow tract obstruction, have been detected so far. This procedure also permits one to correct asymmetric selective dilatations reducing the size of the annulus. At the same time the sphincter-like effect of the mitral orifice, although reduced, is maintained, as observed with echocardiographic short-axis views of the valve. Salati and co-workers[30] utilized metal clips as radiopaque markers when a pericardial tubular prosthesis was utilized for annuloplasty. On fluoroscopic examination they were able to demonstrate preserved variations of size and shape of the mitral orifice throughout cardiac cycle and a systolic reduction of the anteroposterior

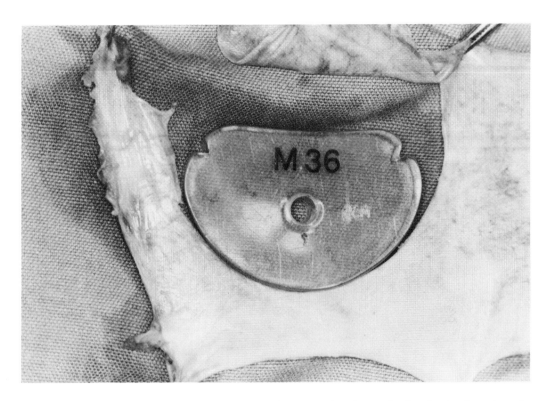

Fig. 8.1. Based on the body surface area of the patient, the appropriate Carpentier ring sizer is selected to tailor the treated autologous pericardial strip utilized to reinforce the annuloplasty.

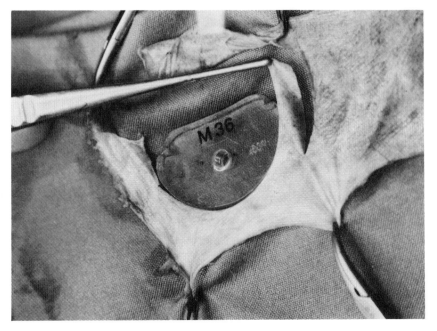

Fig. 8.2. After cutting the inner circumference with a small lancet, parallel incisions are made 0.8 to 1 cm apart with scissors.

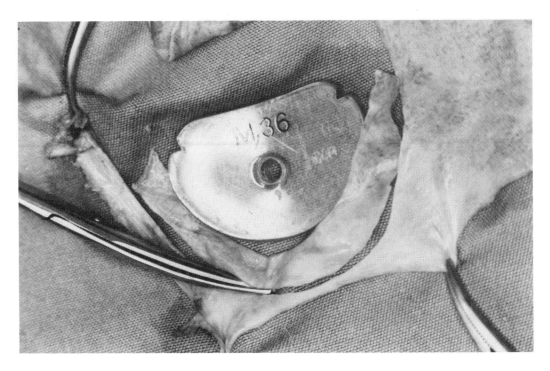

Fig. 8.3. A strip reproducing the shape of the posterior annulus is obtained.

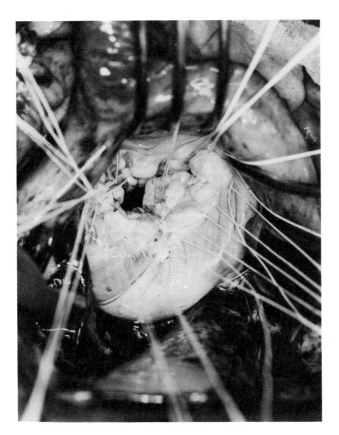

Fig. 8.4. Eight to ten 4-0 Gore-Tex® sutures are anchored in a "U" shape to the posterior annulus from one fibrous trigone to the other with large bites.

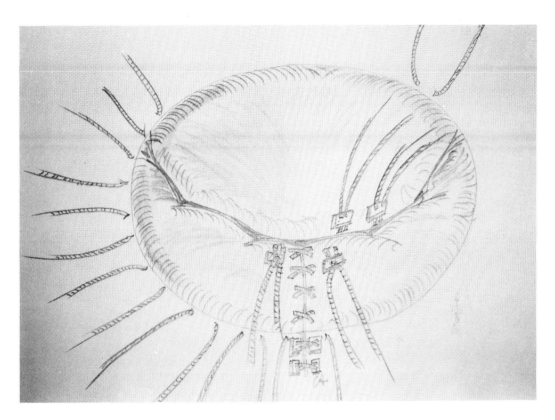

Fig. 8.5. Schematic illustration of the annular stitches placed to perform the pericardium-reinforced annuloplasty.

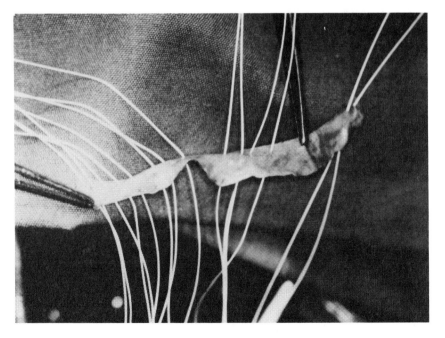

Fig. 8.6. The stitches are then passed close to the inner edge of the strip. The two strands of the same suture are positioned close each other.

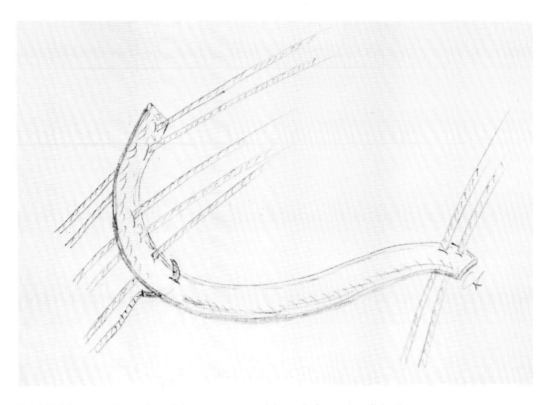

Fig. 8.7. Schematic illustration of the sutures passed through the pericardial strip.

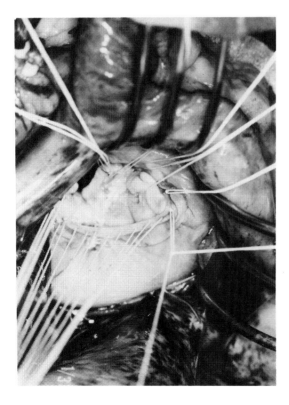

Fig. 8.8. The strip is then laid on the valve annulus so that the smooth surface of pericardium will face blood flow. The stitches are tied.

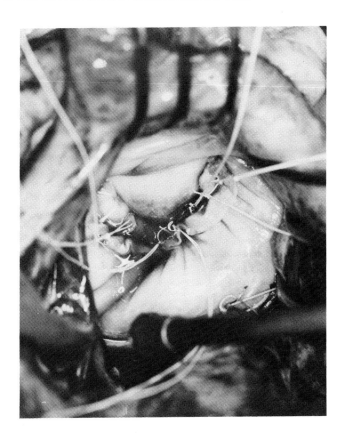

Fig. 8.9. With the ventricle filled with saline solution to close the valve, final adjustment of artificial chordae length is achieved to obtain a symmetric closure line and a satisfactory appositional area. Finally artificial chordae are tied.

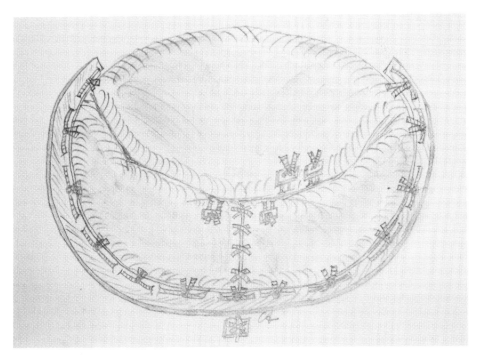

Fig. 8.10. Schematic illustration of the final valve appearance after annuloplasty and artificial chordae tying.

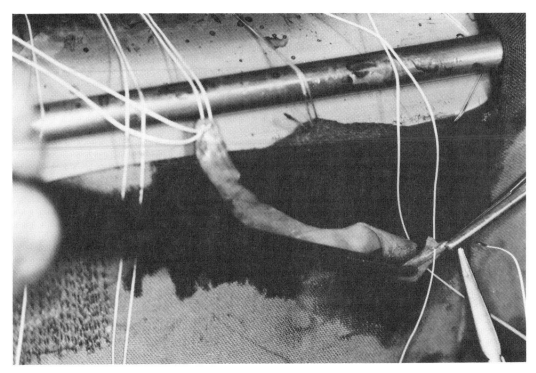

Fig. 8.11. Alternative method to perform a pericardium-reinforced annuloplasty. The extremities of the pericardium strip are secured to the fibrous trigons with two 4-0 Gore-Tex® stitches.

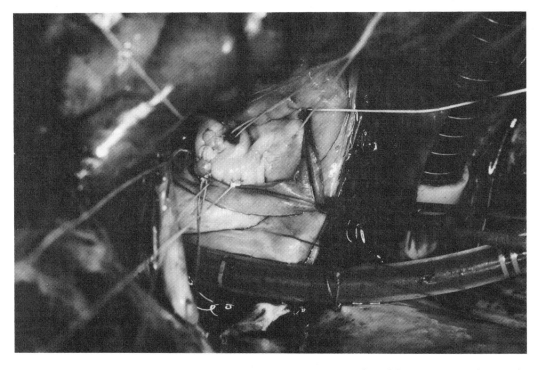

Fig. 8.12. The suture placed on one side is then run to secure the inner edge of the strip to the valve annulus up to the central point.

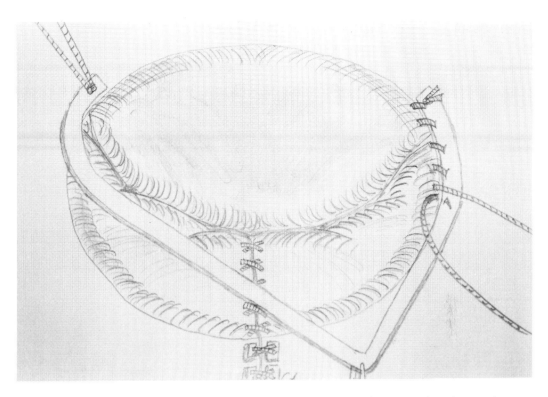

Fig. 8.13. Schematic illustration of the running suture utilized to secure the strip to the valve annulus.

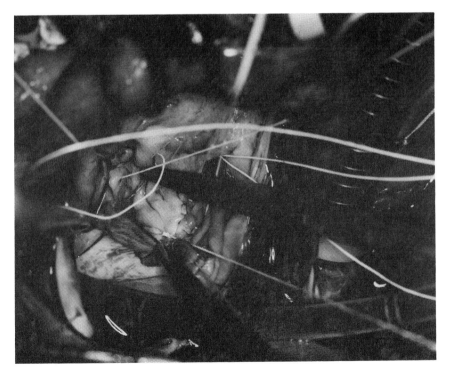

Fig. 8.14. The suture placed on the other trigone is run to reach the central point of the posterior annulus to be tied with the opposite suture.

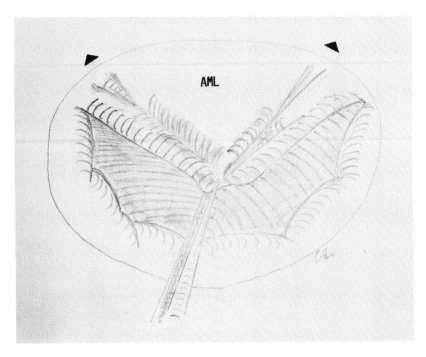

Fig. 8.15. Maneuver utilized to correctly identify the fibrous trigones. Pulling the central part of the anterior leaflet two wrinkles are produced. Their directions toward anterior annulus indicate the sites of the trigones (triangles).

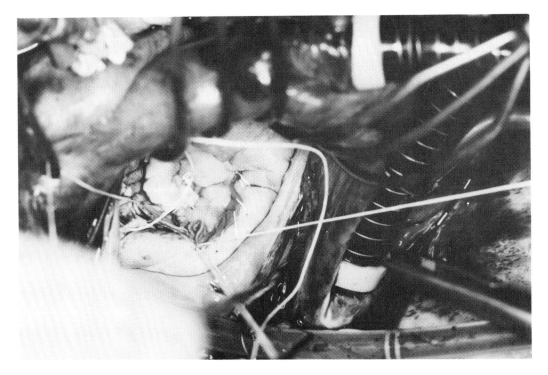

Fig. 8.16. With both techniques of fixation of the inner margin of the strip, the external edge is secured to the atrial wall with a running 4-0 Gore-Tex® suture to obtain a smooth surface.

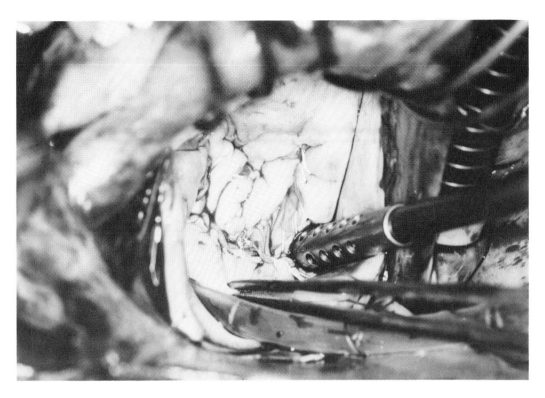

Fig. 8.17. Final appearance of the pericardium-reinforced suture annuloplasty.

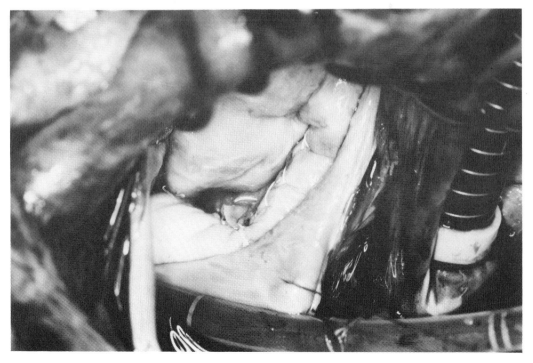

Fig. 8.18. Final hydrodynamic test of the valve demonstrating no regurgitant jets.

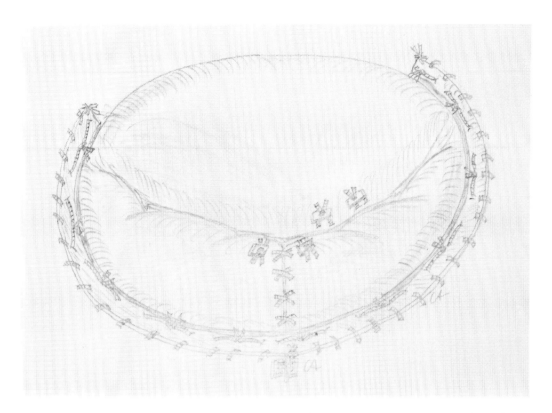

Fig. 8.19. Schematic illustration of the final appearance of a valve reconstructed with artificial chordae, posterior leaflet quadrangular resection and interrupted suture pericardium-reinforced annuloplasty.

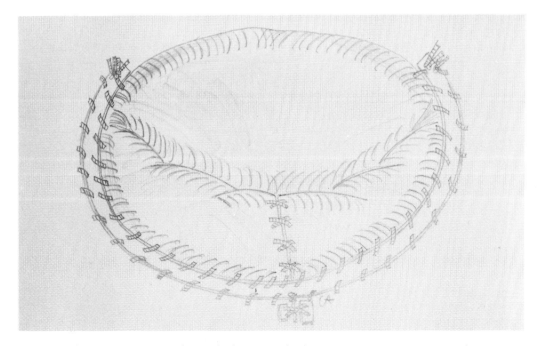

Fig. 8.20. Schematic appearance of a mitral valve repaired utilizing a continuous suture pericardium-reinforced annuloplasty.

diameter of the annulus. These findings were confirmed by echocardiographic examination.

In our experience this technique is safe, effective and reproducible.It requires no artifical ring thereby preventing related complications. Also with echocardiography we confirmed preservation of annular variations during the cardiac cycle and maintenance of normal contractility of the basal segments, usually impaired when rigid devices are utilized. Further investigations will be necessary to confirm these advantages after long-term follow-up.

References

1. Levine RA, Triulzi MO, Harrigan P et al. The relationship of mitral annular shape to the diagnosis of mitral valve prolapse. Circulation 1987; 75:756-67.

2. Davis PKB, Kinmonth JB. The movements of the annulus of the mitral valve. J Cardiovasc Surg 1963; 4:427-31.

3. Spence PA, Peniston CM, David TE et al. Toward a better understanding of the etiology of left ventricular dysfunction after mitral valve replacement: An experimental study with possible clinical implications. Ann Thorac Surg 1986; 41:363-71.

4. Sakai K, Sakaki S, Hirata N et al. Assessment of postoperative left ventricular function after mitral valve repair for mitral regurgitation. Circulation 1991; 84 (Suppl II):II 578.

5. Ormiston JA, Shah PM, Tei C et al. Size and motion of the mitral valve annulus in man. I. A two-dimensional echocardiographic method and findings in normal subjects. Circulation 1981; 64:113-120.

6. van Rijk-Zwikker GL, Mast F, Schipperheyn JJ et al. Comparison of rigid and flexible rings for annulolasty of the porcine mitral valve. Circulation 1990; 82 (Suppl IV):IV 58-IV 64.

7. Handschumacher MD, Sanfilippo AJ, Rodriguez L et al. Dynamic three-dimensional echocardiographic reconstruction of the normal human mitral valve. Circulation 1990; 82 (Suppl III):III 69.

8. Wooler GH, Nixon PGF, Grimshaw VA et al. Experience with repair of the mitral valve in mitral incompetence. Thorax 1962; 17:49-57.

9. Kay JH, Egerton WS. The repair of mitral insufficiency associated with ruptured chordae tendineae. Ann Surg 1963; 157:351-60.

10. Reed GE, Pooley RW, Moggio RA. Durability of measured mitral annuloplasty. Seventeen-year study. J Thorac Cardiovasc Surg 1980; 79:321-5.

11. Shore DF, Wong P, Paneth M. Results of mitral valvuloplasty with a suture plication technique. J Thorac Cardiovasc Surg 1980; 79:349-57.

12. Carpentier A, Chauvaud S, Fabiani JN et al. Reconstructive surgery of mitral incompetence. Ten-year appraisal. J Thorac Cardiovasc Surg 1980; 79:338-48.

13. Duran CMG, Pomar JL, Cucchiara G. A Flexible ring for atrioventricular heart valve reconstruction. J Cardiovasc Surg 1978; 19:417-20.

14. Duran CG. Valve reconstruction for rheumatic mitral disease with the Duran ring. Semin Thorac Cardiovasc Surg 1989; 1:176-82.

15. Puig Massana M, Calbet JM, Castells E. Conservative surgery of the mitral valve. Annuloplasty on a new adjustable ring. In: Birks W, Ostermeyer J, Schults HD, eds. Proceedings of the 29th International Congress of the European Society of Cardiovascular Surgery. New York: Springer-Verlag, 1981:30-7.

16. Gorton ME, Piehler JM, Killen DA et al. Mitral valve repair using a flexible and adjustable annuloplasty ring. Ann Thorac Surg 1993; 55:860-3.

17. Duran C. Evolution of the techniques of annuloplasty. Proceedings of Medtronic Cardiovascular Technology Symposium. Ayrshire, Scotland, October 24-27,1991.

18. David TE, Komeda M, Pollick C et al. Mitral valve annuloplasty: The effect of the type on left ventricular function. Ann Thorac Surg 1989; 47:524-8.

19. David TE. Effect of mitral annuloplasty ring in left ventricular function. Semin Thorac Cardiovasc Surg 1989; 1:144-8.

20. Rayhill SC, Castro LJ, Nizyporuk MA et al. Rigid ring fixation of the mitral annulus does not impair left ventricular systolic function in the normal canine heart. Circulation

1992; 86 (Suppl II):II 26-II 38.

21. Sakai K, Nakano S, Taniguchi K et al. Global left ventricular performance and regional systolic function after suture annuloplasty for chronic mitral regurgitation. Circulation 1992; 86 (Suppl II):II 39-II 45.

22. Czer LSC, Maurer G, Trento A et al. Comparative efficacy of ring and suture annuloplasty for ischemic mitral regurgitation. Circulation 1992; 86 (Suppl II):II 46-II 52.

23. Lee KS, Stewart WJ, Lever HM et al. Mechanism of outflow tract obstruction causing failed mitral valve repair: Anterior displacement of leaflet coaptation. Circulation 1992; 86 (Suppl I):I 496.

24. Jebara VA, Mihaileanu SA, Acar C et al. Can left ventricular outflow obstruction be avoided after mitral valve repair: Results of a new surgical technique. Circulation 1992; 86 (Suppl I):I 496.

25. Deloche A, Jebara VA, Relland JYM et al. Valve repair with Carpentier techniques. The second decade. J Thorac Cardiovasc Surg 1990; 99:990-1002.

26. Wilson JH, Rath R, Glaser R et al. Severe hemolysis after incomplete mitral valve repair. Ann Thorac Surg 1990; 50:136-7.

27. Dilip KA, Vachaspathy P, Clarke B et al. Haemolysis following mitral valve repair. J Cardiovasc Surg 1992; 33:568-9.

28. David TE, Bos J, Rakowski H. Mitral valve repair by replacement of chordae tendineae with polytetrafluoroethylene sutures. J Thorac Cardiovasc Surg 1991; 101:495-501.

29. David TE, Feindel CM. Reconstruction of the mitral annulus. Circulation 1987; 76 (3 Pt 2):III 102-III 107.

30. Salati M, Scrofani R, Santoli C. Posterior pericardial annuloplasty: A physiological correction? Eur J Cardio-thorac Surg 1991; 5:226-9.

31. Hendren WG, Nemec JJ, Lytle BW et al. Mitral valve repair for ischemic mitral insufficiency. Ann Thorac Surg 1991; 52:1246-52.

32. Salvador L, Rocco F, Ius P et al. The pericardium reinforced suture annuloplasty: Another tool available for mitral annulus repair? J Card Surg 1993; 8:79-84.

CHAPTER 9

ECHOCARDIOGRAPHY FOR ARTIFICIAL CHORDAE INSERTION

Echocardiographic findings in cases of mitral valve reconstruction are of more value to cardiac surgeons than are hemodynamic data obtained by cardiac catheterization. Indeed two-dimensional and color Doppler echocardiography provide morphologic and functional information about valve motion and dysfunction of ventricular wall, papillary muscles, chordae tendineae, mitral leaflets and annulus. Moreover epicardial and transesophageal echocardiography have significantly improved image quality, particularly with regard to the subvalvular apparatus, which often requires special attention during mitral valve repair. Stewart and Salcedo[1] have written that echocardiography is for the surgeon performing valve repair what coronary arteriography is for the surgeon performing coronary grafting. They suggested a systematic approach[2] to mitral valve analysis similar to that suggested by Carpentier.[3]

Echocardiography represents the conjunction of the different components of the diagnostic and therapeutic teams: cardiologists, surgeons and anesthesiologists.[1] Accurate transesophageal echocardiographic examination plays a significant role in several phases of the treatment of mitral valve disease.

First, evaluation of anatomical and functional abnormalities of the components of the mitral apparatus from the ventricular wall to the annulus is crucial in predicting repair outcome. Cormier and co-workers[4] compared preoperative transthoracic and transesophageal echocardiographic findings in mitral regurgitation with surgical findings with respect to the type of lesion, mechanism, etiology and the choice of surgical procedure (valve repair versus replacement). They found that transthoracic echocardiography has a sensitivity of 86% in the evaluation of the etiology. The mechanism of the regurgitation was correctly predicted in most cases with the exception of chordal rupture, which could be demonstrated preoperatively only in 30% of the cases. On the other hand transesophageal echocardiography was 100% accurate in determining etiology. Chordal rupture was determined in all but one case. Both techniques were able to predict the type of surgical procedure in more than 85% of the cases.

The superiority of transesophageal to transthoracic echocardiography in demonstrating anatomic abnormalities of the mitral valve, including ruptured chordae tendineae, has been reported also by Alam and co-workers.[5] Similar findings have been reported by Hozumi and co-workers.[6] They found that transesophageal echocardiography has a sensitivity of 100% in detecting ruptured chordae, compared with 35% of transthoracic echocardiography. Yet both techniques have a specificity of 100%; both revealed no chordal abnormalities in patients without chordal rupture.

Two recent studies focused on the role of Doppler color flow mapping of mitral valve regurgitation in flail mitral leaflet.[7,8] Pearson and co-workers[7] described the typical direction of the regurgitant jet with regard to the leaflet involved. With posterior flail leaflet, this direction is along the posterior surface of the anterior leaflet toward the posterior wall of the aorta. This jet is highly eccentric and turbulent, making underestimation of severe mitral regurgitation likely. On the other hand in some cases this jet is easier to determine than the flail portion of the leaflet itself. In anterior flail leaflet a jet directed toward the posterolateral atrial wall was always clearly detected. It is usually large and less turbulent. Also the authors quantified the severity of mitral regurgitation based on two different parameters since the most appropriate method is yet established. They utilized both absolute jet area and jet area/left atrial area observing that in the presence of flail leaflet, particularly when it is posterior, these parameters easily underestimate the severity of regurgitation. Therefore the authors suggested the use of pulsed Doppler ultrasound with color flow mapping to calculate the regurgitant fraction not influenced by the type of lesion in cases with suspected flail leaflet and suspected underestimation of the degree of regurgitation .

A new method for quantitative assessment of regurgitant volume by color Doppler echocardiography was developed by Tanabe and co-workers.[9] They calculated this value by deducing left ventricular outflow volume from mitral inflow volume, and they found that this value significantly correlates with that obtained with ultrafast computed tomography.

Another experimental method to quantify mitral regurgitation was clinically tested by Chen and co-workers.[10] It utilized proximal isovelocity surface area. They found that this method positively correlates with the severity of mitral regurgitation, when com-

pared with angiographic data unless a very large regurgitant jet is present, making likely underestimation of the insufficiency.

Himelman and co-workers,[8] besides confirming the characteristics of the regurgitant jet in cases of flail mitral leaflets, introduced a new parameter to validate the diagnosis with transesophageal echocardiography. They calculated the ratio of jet arc length to jet arc radius of curvatureand found a significant correlation between a ratio >2.5 and the presence of flail leaflet. With eccentric jets, in the absence of flail leaflet, this ratio was < 2.5, whereas it was always >2.5 when a flail leaflet was demonstrated.

The influence of jet direction on pulmonary venous flow pattern in cases of severe mitral regurgitation was addressed by Pearson and co-workers[11] with transesophageal echocardiography. Since the direction and velocity of mid-systolic pulmonary venous flow may indicate the severity of mitral regurgitation, they evaluated how regurgitant jet direction influences reversal of flow. They found that direction (medial, lateral or central) does not influence mid-systolic flow reversal, so this could be a significant indicator of the severity of mitral regurgitation.

Preoperative echocardiography for the prediction of repair outcome was evaluated by Perinetti et al.[12] Starting from the consideration that this technique was particularly sensitive in predicting the prolapse of each component of the valve, they classified patients in four groups based on this pathological element. They found that when the posterior leaflet is involved alone, there is a significantly higher probability of valve repair when compared with patients with prolapse of the anterior or both leaflets.

Another mechanism producing severe mitral regurgitation, besides chordal rupture, was described by Fraser et al.[13] The asymmetric apposition of leaflets in the presence of intact systolic coaptation along the entire line of closure proved to be sufficient by itself to determine severe mitral regurgitation when it exceeds 3 mm, since the minimum depth of normal apposition was found to be 2.9 ±0.3 mm in normal hearts. The authors echocardiographically evaluated patients with severe mitral regurgitation without any prolapse of the body of the leaflet; they found a mean abnormal apposition of 4.9 ± 0.2 mm. This echocardiographic evidence may help in identifying candidates for mitral reconstruction.

Another area in which echocardiography serves as an important tool for cardiac surgeons is intraoperative evaluation of patients treated with mitral valve repair. Epicardial and biplane transesophageal echocardiographic examination, before cardiopulmonary by-pass is initiated, offers to the surgeon a superb anatomic view of the valve components so that he can identify the site and degree of the lesions. In our experience this is very accurate ain identifying the areas of true prolapse of the leaflets in a normally beating heart. Yet interpretation of the echocardiographic findings,without visual inspection of the valve after opening a flaccid arrested heart, is not completely satisfactory. In the presence of certain reference points, such as the posterior leaflet area near the anterolateral commissure that is rarely involved in degenerative pathology,[3,14] traction applied to the subvalvular apparatus may produce misleading results, mostly in the presence of redundant anterior leaflets. In particular echocardiography distinguises true anterior leaflet prolapse produced by chordae elongation or rupture from the free margin arising above the annular plane from the upward displacement of the appositional area of the leaflet produced by loss of coaptation due to flail posterior leaflet and/or annular dilatation, with the free margin of the anterior leaflet maintained below the annular plane.

The second intraoperative application of echocardiography occurs early after weaning the patient from cardiopulmonary by-pass. This permits one to verify the result obtained with open-heart hydrodynamic tests, to reestablish cardiopulmonary bypass, and to perform further valve procedures (repair or replacement) in case echocardiographic findings are not satisfactory. In our experience this has been the case in 1 of 107 patients, while the hydrodynamic test indicated the need for valve replacement in 3 patients.

Sheikh et al[15] reported unsatisfactory results requiring immediate further surgery in 10 (6%) of their patients. De Simone et al[16] analyzed their experience with intraoperative transesophageal echocardiography finding that this technique is an ideal diagnostic tool for assessing the adequacy of valve repair, provided the surgeons are well-trained in making decisions based on this technique.

The role of contrast echocardiography (saline solution injection into the ventricular cavity) was studied by Viossat et al.[17] The results obtained with this method when performed before cardiopulmonary bypass closely correlated with the preoperative evaluation. After valve repair the patients could be classified in three groups: those with absent or minimal regurgitation (12/20), those with moderate regurgitation (5/20) and those in which a marked regurgitation (3/20) suggested prompt resumption of cardiopulmonary by-pass to improve the repair (two cases) or to replace the valve (one case).

The correlation between intraoperative transesophageal echocardiographic findings after mitral valve repair and the angiographic determination of residual regurgitation observed several weeks after the procedure was evaluated by Reichert et al.[18] They found a good correlation between the two methods ($r=0.83$; $p<0.001$). In their experience before this study, they reported two cases of severe residual mitral regurgitation in whom the valve was not replaced during the same procedure because the traditional hydrodynamic test in the arrested heart was satisfactory and transesophageal echocardiography did not demonstrate a regurgitant jet.

A different conclusion were drawn by Moulijn et al.[19] They compared the results obtained by open-heart hydrodynamic testing and those of intraoperative transesophageal echocardiography to postoperative left ventricular angiography. They could not find any significant difference in reliability between results obtained with hydrodynamic testing and echocardiography with regard to residual regurgitation.

Assoun et al[20] utilized intraoperative transesophageal echocardiography to predict residual mitral regurgitation. Among the parameters analyzed, they found that the absolute leaflet coaptation length and this value normalized for the total length of the leaflets are two measures significantly inversely correlated with the degree of residual regurgitation after mitral valve repair.

Another application of intraoperative echocardiography is evaluation of ventricular function. Goldman et al[21] compared the intraoperative effects of valve repair versus replacement. They observed significant global and regional ventricular dysfunction after traditional valve replacement with papillary muscle-annular discontinuity, with concomitant reduction of ejection fraction. On the other hand myocardial contractility was preserved after valve repair. The authors emphasized the value of intraoperative echocardiography as a means of obtaining an immediate, reliable evaluation of the results. This should encourage surgeons to attempt valve repair in any case of mitral regurgitation.

The third application of echocardiography is for follow-up. In our experience, during the early learning phase of a new technique, such as artificial chordae insertion, it is essential for the surgeon himself to "visually" inspect the behavior of the repaired valve to improve surgical technique and recognize possible early signs of malfunction. In particular, ventricular function, subvalvular apparatus abnormalities, leaflet motion, leaflet tissue quality, leaflet retraction and annular dilatation should be checked. Obviously any sign of valve malfunction, although hemodynamically insignificant, should be followed to prevent sudden deterioration and to perform reoperation, if required.

In our experience, in order to follow a new surgical technique, in the absence of any clinical sign of valve malfunction, one transthoracic echocardiographic evaluation every six months and one transesophageal evaluation every year should be performed.

ECHOCARDIOGRAPHY FOR ARTIFICIAL CHORDAE INSERTION

Most of the questions regarding preoperative echocardiography of the patients scheduled for mitral valve repair are common to every type of procedure utilized. However insertion of artificial chordae requires careful attention to a few aspects from the cardiac surgeon's point of view in particular (Table 9.1).

1. Is the movement of the leaflet normal, reduced or increased? Following the introduction of Carpentier's functional approach,[22] this observation immediately discloses the type of lesion affecting the valve. In mitral regurgitation and normal leaflet motion, isolated annular dilatation or leaflet perforation should be responsible for the insufficiency. When leaflet motion is restricted this can result from chordal pathology, such as fusion, or leaflet pathology, such as thickening and/or commissural fusion. Increased leaflet motion, producing prolapse, may be caused by chordal or papillary muscle elongation or rupture.

2. Is only one leaflet or are both leaflets involved? As already mentioned, it is essential to distinguish "billowing", in which excessive leaflet tissue creates a dome into the atrium during systole but the free margin is maintained below the annular plane, from real "prolapse," in which the free margin rises above the annular plain (Fig. 9.1 and 9.2). It is also very important to distinguish the prolapse, in which subvalvular apparatus anomalies should be corrected, from the upward displacement of the coaptation area due to inadequate apposition to the corresponding part of the contralateral leaflet (Fig. 9.2), in which the procedure should be restricted to restore normal coaptation. Careful scan of the leaflets from the anterolateral to the posteromedial commissures should be performed to define all areas of abnormal leaflet motion to prevent incomplete correction based only on the visual, flaccid open-heart inspection.

3. Which chordae are elongated or broken? Related to the previous point is analysis of specific chordal pathology. It is crucial to carefully inspect all chordae, including the commissural ones, to correct all areas of pathology.

4. What is the condition of the subvalvular apparatus, besides the chordae? This evaluation should include ventricular wall and papillary muscles. Indeed paradoxical motion of the area of insertion of the papillary muscles may produce, if not diagnosed in the beating heart, an unsatisfactory repair. This problem sometimes goes unrecognized in hydro-

Table 1. Echocardiographic examination for artificial chordae insertion

*Preoperative Evaluation
1. Is the movement of the leaflets normal, reduced or increased?
2. Is only one leaflet interested or are they both involved?
3. Which chordae are elongated or broken?
4. Situation of the subvalvular apparatus, besides chordae.
5. Characteristics of the regurgitant flow.
6. Annular dilatation.

*Intraoperative Evaluation after Valve Repair
1. Residual regurgitation.
2. Iatrogenic mitral stenosis.
3. Left ventricular outflow tract obstruction.
4. Basic morphologic characteristics of artificial chordae.

dynamic testing in the arrested heart.

This happened in one of our mitral repairs without chordal insertion and required valve replacement. Transesophageal echocardiography performed after cardiopulmonary by-pass to determine signs of mitral regurgitation demonstrated anomalous paradoxical motion of the area of insertion of the posteromedial papillary muscle in the absence of ischemic pathology.

5. What are the characteristics of the regurgitant flow: direction, extension, relevance and duration? It is important to confirm the observations performed on the leaflets. The direction of the jet is usually toward the non-involved leaflet (Fig. 9.1). If it is central this can be due to prolapse of both leaflets or to annular dilatation with loss of coaptation of leaflets (Fig. 9.2). The extension of the regurgitant flow over the plane of the valve annulus in the short axis indicates the area in which the surgeon should restore leaflet coaptation. This view also reveals if multiple jets are present. The relevance of regurgitant flow is indicated by its extension into the left atrium and by reversal flow into the pulmonary veins. Also duration during systole is an index of the severity of the lesion.

6. Is the annulus dilated? Since annuloplasty should be performed in the great majority of valve repairs, it is relevant to evaluate the degree of dilatation of the annulus (Fig. 9.1 and 9.2). This is particularly useful when a suture annuloplasty is planned to correct reduction of the annulus. On intraoperative epicardial or transesophageal echocardiography some additional aspects should be carefully checked as well.

1. Residual regurgitation. While a trivial regurgitant jet is quite acceptable after mitral valve repair (Fig. 9.3), mild to moderate regurgitation should be carefully evaluated to determine if further procedures on the valve (repair or replacement) are indicated. In particular, the type, duration and direction of regurgitant flow should be defined. From the length of the jet into the left atrium and its extension on the transverse plan, one can establish the severity of insufficiency. In addition the flow into the pulmonary veins indicates, when reversed, severe, unacceptable residual regurgitation. Moreover the degree of insufficiency can be quantified from the duration through systole of the regurgitant flow. In fact, a very short central protosystolic jet is often seen, mostly in very redundant or fibrotic valves with possible increased closure inertia (Fig. 9.3). This is more common soon after cardiopulmonary by-pass and particularly when drugs, such as isoproterenol, are utilized. In our experience this type of jet is quite acceptable. It does not correspond to significant hemodynamic dysfunction. Often it decreases in 24 hours, disappearing in more than 50% of cases before hospital discharge.

The direction of the jet should be accurately investigated for two main reasons. First, from the direction the surgeon can ascertain the cause of residual regurgitation facilitating an additional reparative procedure, if required. Second, clinically significant hemolysis[22-24] may also be produced by a small jet if it is directed against a prosthetic ring or an artificial pledget.

All these observations are very useful. In degenerative valve disease we observed stable findings throughout the follow-up, while in rheumatic cases the recurrence of mitral regurgitation with progressive increase of the degree of insufficiency was found in 7 out of 19 patients.

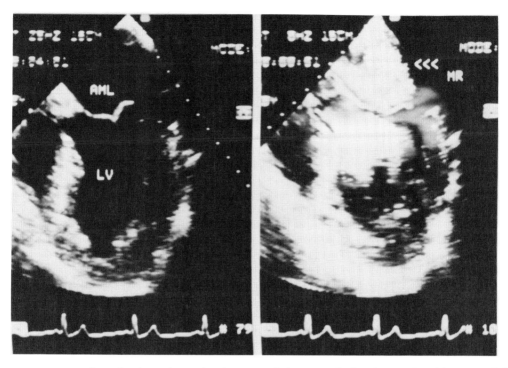

Fig. 9.1. Transesophageal echocardiography showing a flail anterior leaflet due to chordal rupture (left), producing massive mitral regurgitation demonstrated by 2-D color Doppler echocardiography (right). Annular dilatation is evident as well. AML=anterior mitral leaflet; LV=left ventricle; MR=mitral regurgitant jet.

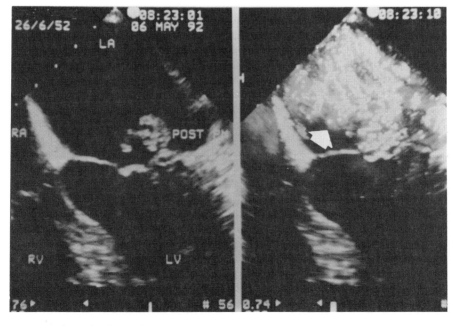

Fig. 9.2. Transesophageal echocardiography showing a flail posterior mitral leaflet due to chordal rupture (left), producing massive mitral regurgitation (arrow) demonstrated 2-D color Doppler echocardiography (right).

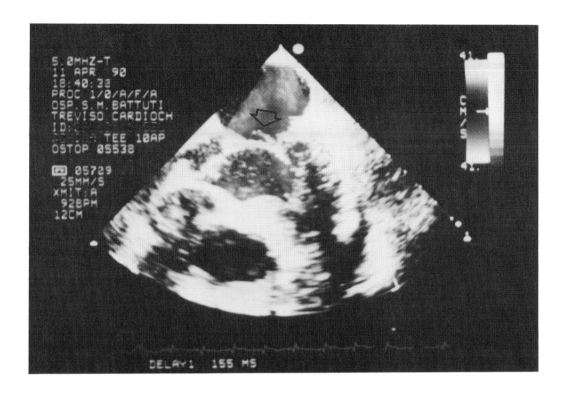

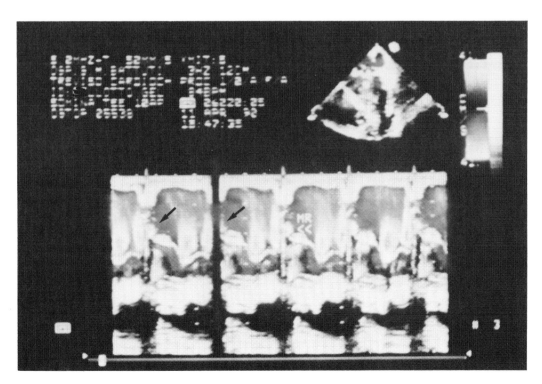

Fig. 9.3 A and B. Trivial residual regurgitant jet (arrow) after valve repair without any hemodynamic significance (A). M-mode color Doppler echocardiography confirms the insignificance of the regurgitant jet (arrows) that is confined to protosystole. MR=mitral regurgitant jet.

2. *Iatrogenic mitral stenosis.* Suture annuloplasty, although performed, with our technique, over a strip of pericardium tailored with a Carpentier ring sizer, may produce excessive tightening of the annulus. In our experience, only one case treated with simple suture annuloplasty without pericardial reinforcement had a restrictive orifice, 1.8 cm^2.

3. *Another possible complication associated with annuloplasty is left ventricular outflow tract obstruction produced by the utilization of a prosthetic ring.*[25-28] In our experience of applying Carpentier rings, although limited, we didn't encounter this complication.

4. *Finally postoperative echocardiography should be used to collect baseline findings regarding e-PTFE chordae and pericardium-reinforced suture annuloplasty.* Since no long-term follow-up is available yet for any of this techniques, it is relevant to establish the"normal" appearance of these structures. Artificial chordae appear as rectilinear structures, thicker and more refractive than natural chordae, although they are really thinner (Fig. 9.4). Also pericardial pledgets appear as thick, homogeneous elements more refractive than papillary muscles (Fig 9.5 and 9.6). The pericardial strip reinforcing the suture annuloplasty can be followed from one trigone to the other (Fig. 9.7) along the posterior annulus (Fig. 9.8). It has been shown that it crimps in accordance with the cardiac cycle and allows the circumferential basal muscular fibers of the ventricle to contract in systole, contrary to the effect produced by the application of rigid rings. Also prosthetic rings can be easily visualized in this phase (Fig. 9.6). So far in serial echocardiographic examinations up to 80 months for artificial chordae and up to 48 months for autologous pericardium-reinforced suture annuloplasty, we could not find any signs of significant modifications, thickening or calcification, of the artificial structures (Fig 9.9).

In recurrent regurgitation, with the exception of two patients that were reoperated, artificial chordae seem to retain the original length, and the insufficiency—all in cases of rheumatic etiology—appears correlated instead with the progression of leaflet shrinkage.

Detachment of artificial chordae from papillary insertion has been observed, as reported by David et al.[22] Artificial chordae have been shownto be under tension throughout cardiac cycle, as natural chordae. Their systolic-diastolic arc of rotation at the site of origin from the papillary muscle appeared unchanged in follow-up, allowing wide excursion of the leaflets. Longer follow-up will be necessary to prove if echocardiographic examinations will be able to discover early signs of artificial chordae degeneration or annuloplasty alterations.

For all these reasons echocardiography is an essential tool in "modern" mitral valve repair. Besides the obvious diagnostic value in all phases of the treatment of valve disease, it is very helpful for surgeons working to improve techniques and increase self confidence. The indications for valve repair broaden with the use of echocardiography, since results can be ascertained immediately and, if necessary, valves replaced promptly. Now almost all patients with mitral regurgitation can be treated operatively.

REFERENCES

1. Stewart WJ, Salcedo EE. Echocardiography in patients undergoing mitral valve surgery. Semin Thorac Cardiovasc Surg 1989; 1:194.

2. Stewart WJ, Agler DA, Homa DA et al. Predicting the mechanism of mitral regurgitation prior to repair: A system using leaflet motion and color Doppler jet direction. Circulation 1990; 82 (Suppl III):III 551.

3. Carpentier A. Cardiac valve surgery—the "French correction." J Thorac Cardiovasc Surg 1983; 86:323-37.

4. Cormier B, Starkman C, Enriquez-Sarano et al. L'echographie des insuffisances mitrales chirurgicales. Diagnostic lesionnel et prevision du type de chirurgie. Arch Mal Coeur 1990; 83:345-50.

5. Alam M, Sun I. Superiority of transesophageal echocardiography in detecting ruptured mitral chordae tendineae. Am Heart J 1991; 121:1819-21.

6. Hozumi T, Yoshikawa J, Yoshida K et al. Direct visualization of ruptured chordae tendineae by transesophageal two-dimensional echocardiography. J Am Coll Cardiol

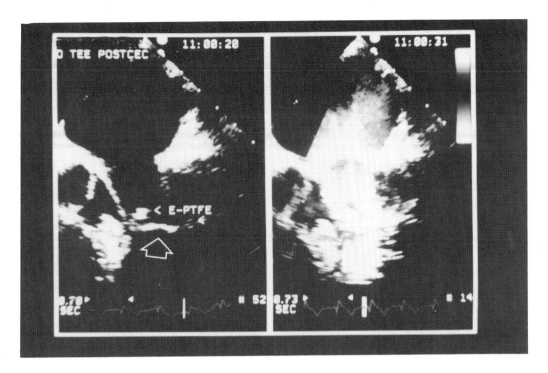

Fig. 9.4. Appearance of "normal" artificial chordae soon after implantation (arrow). They appear thicker and more refractive than natural chordae, although they are thinner. Diastolic phase. e-PTFE=artificial chordae.

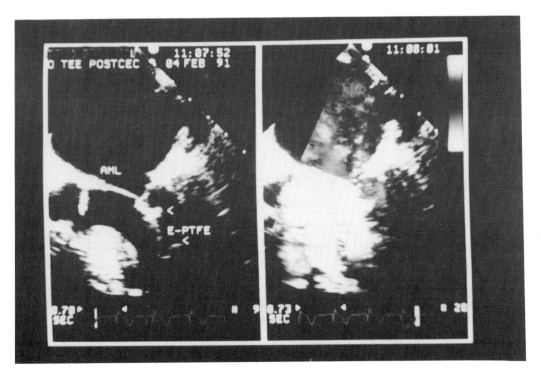

Fig. 9.5. Autologous pericardial pledgets (arrows) appear more refractive than papillary muscles. Systolic phase. AML=anterior mitral leaflet; e-PTFE=artificial chorda.

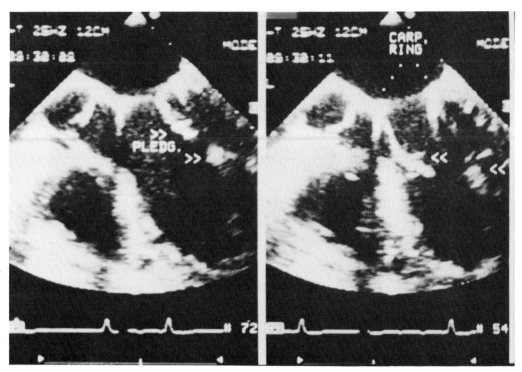

Fig. 9.6. In some cases only pericardial pledgets appear (arrows) as refractive structures, while artificial chordae are not evident. PLEDG=pericardial pledgets; CARP RING=Carpentier ring.

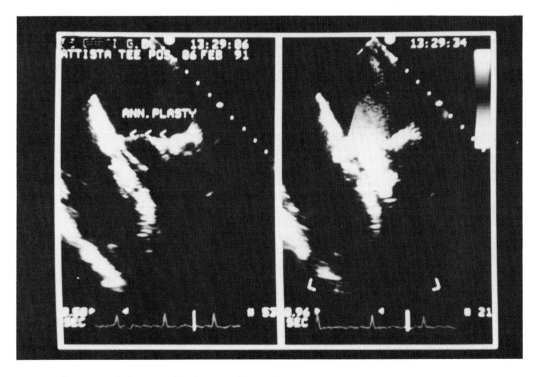

Fig. 9.7. The pericardial strip utilized to reinforce the annuloplasty is evident near the posteromedial commissure (arrows).

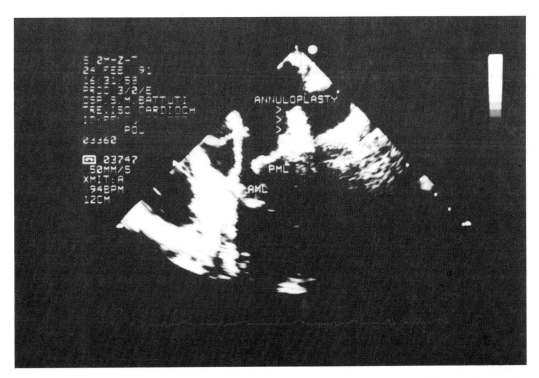

Fig. 9.8. The same pericardial strip appears as a wide refractive structure in corresponding to the posterior annulus, extending to the atrial wall (arrows).

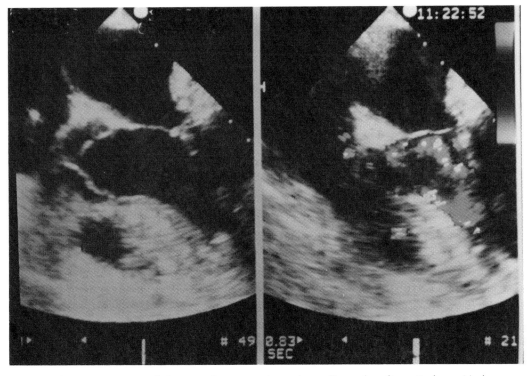

Fig. 9.9. The same patient of Figure 5 (intraoperative echocardiography after mitral repair) shows no modifications of artificial chordae appearance 52 months later.

1990; 16:1315-9.

7. Pearson AC, St. Vrain J, Mrosek D et al. Color Doppler echocardiographic evaluation of patients with a flail mitral leaflet. J Am Coll Cardiol 1990; 16:232-9.

8. Himelman RB, Kusumoto F, Oken K et al. The flail mitral valve: Echocardiographic findings by precordial and transesophageal imaging and Doppler color flow mapping. J Am Coll Cardiol 1991; 17:272-9.

9. Tanabe K, Yamagishi M, Nakatani S et al. A new method for quantitative assessment of regurgitant volume of isolated mitral insufficiency by color Doppler echocardiography. Circulation 1990; 82 (Suppl III):III 552.

10. Chen C, Koschyk D, Mehl C et al. Comparison of quantifying mitral regurgitation using color Doppler proximal isovelocity surface area and angiography. Circulation 1991; 84 (Suppl II):II 637.

11. Pearson AC, Alton ME, Whyles RJ et al. Jet direction does not effect pulmonary venous flow reversal in left and right pulmonary veins in severe mitral regurgitation. Circulation 1991; 84 (Suppl II):II 105.

12. Perinetti M, De Gevigney G, Delahaye F et al. L'echocardiographie dans la selection des malades avant valvuloplastie mitrale de Carpentier. Arch Mal Coeur 1990; 83:53-61.

13. Fraser AG, McAlpine HM, Chow L et al. Abnormal apposition as the cause of mitral regurgitation in patients with intact leaflet coaptation. Circulation 1990; 82 (Suppl III):III 241.

14. Cosgrove DM. Mitral valve repair in patients with elongated chordae tendineae. J Cardiac Surg 1989; 4:247-52.

15. Sheikh K, DeBrujin, Rankin JS et al. The utility of transesophageal echocardiography and Doppler color flow imaging in patients undergoing cardiac valve surgery. J Am Coll Cardiol 1990; 15:363-72.

16. De Simone R, Lange R, Saggau W et al. Intraoperative transesophageal echocardiography for the evaluation of mitral, aortic and tricuspid valve repair. A tool to optimize surgical outcome. Eur J Cardio-thorac Surg 1992; 6:665-73.

17. Viossat J, Chauvaud S, Mihaileanu S et al.

Evaluation per-operatoire de la plastie mitral par l'echocardiographie bidimensionnelle de contraste. Arch Mal Coeur 1986; 79:1475-9.

18. Reichert SLA, Visser CA, Moulijn AC et al. Intraoperative transesophageal color-coded Doppler echocardiography for evaluation of residual regurgitation after mitral valve repair. J Thorac Cardiovasc Surg 1990; 100:756-61.

19. Moulijn AC, Smulders YM, Koolen JJ et al. Intraoperative assessment of the mitral valve: Transesophageal Doppler echocardiography vs left ventricular filling on the flaccid heart. Eur J Cardio-thorac Surg 1992; 6:122-6.

20. Assoun B, Diebold B, Abergel E et al. Morphology-function relationship after mitral valve repair. Circulation 1992; 86 (Suppl I):I 724.

21. Goldman ME, Mora F, Guarino T et al. Mitral valvuloplasty is superior to valve replacement for preservation of left ventricular function: An intraoperative two-dimensional echocardiographic study. J Am Coll Cardiol 1987; 10:568-75.

22. David TE, Bos J, Rakowski H. Mitral valve repair by replacement of chordae tendineae with polytetrafluoroethylene sutures. J Thorac Cardiovasc Surg 1991; 101:495-501.

23. Wilson JH, Rath R, Glaser R et al. Severe hemolysis after incomplete mitral valve repair. Ann Thorac Surg 1990; 50:136-7.

24. Dilip KA, Vachaspathy P, Clarke B et al. Haemolysis following mitral valve repair. J Cardiovasc Surg 1992; 33:568-9.

25. Kreindel MS, Schiavone WA, Lever HM et al. Systolic anterior motion of the mitral valve after Carpentier ring valvuloplasty for mitral valve prolapse. Am J Cardiol 1986; 57:408-12.

26. Carpentier A. The S.A.M. issue. "Le Club Mitrale" Newsletter. 1989; 1:5.

27. Carpentier A. The sliding leaflet technique. "Le Club Mitrale" Newsletter 1988; 1:5.

28. Deloche A, Jebara VA, Relland JYM et al. Valve repair with Carpentier techniques. The second decade. J Thorac Cardiovasc Surg 1990; 99:990-1002.

CHAPTER 10

ROLE OF THE SUBVALVULAR APPARATUS IN MITRAL VALVE REPLACEMENT

At the sixty-ninth Meeting of the American Association for Thoracic Surgery, held in Boston in 1989, C. Walton Lillehei[1] recalled three papers published by himself and his colleagues in 1963 and 1964[2] in which they recommended preserving as much as possible of the subvalvular apparatus during mitral valve replacement (MVR). In his experience with preservation, the incidence of postoperative low output syndrome fell and operative mortality decreased from 37% to 14%. Traditional MVR technique involves complete disconnection of the mitral annulus from the papillary muscles which results in increased afterload due to the elimination of the "low resistance regurgitant jet" and reduced left ventricular (LV) ejection fraction due to the abolition of the favorable function of the subvalvular apparatus on LV function.[3-9] And in a recent editorial, Carabello[10] affirmed that there is no more doubt about the importance of chordal preservation in MVR. In fact preservation of the subvalvular apparatus permits surgery in patients with poor ventricular function. Yet these conclusions come only after many years of controversy regarding the preservation of the subvalvular apparatus.

In the early '60s Lillehei's suggestion was not accepted widely and was even thought dangerous by some surgeons. Presumably this was due to contemporaneous reports by Bjork et al[11] and Rastelli[12] et al that did not demonstrate any advantage of preservation of the subvalvular apparatus. The inadequate methods to evaluate the efficacy of the technique may probably account for these results. Bjork et al[11] based theirconclusions mainly on hemodynamic parameters, which do not adequately reflect improvements in left ventricular (LV) function after surgery. Rastelli et al[12] evaluated only cardiac output and filling pressure in a canine model and the lack of significant differences may be due to the dependence of these variables on other physiological parameters. On the other hand, other authors found significant variations only in cardiac output among different groups of patients, when hemodynamic data were analyzed.[13-15]

After 20 years of isolated reports,[16,17] in 1983 David[18] and Hetzer[19] reintroduced Lillehei's suggestion, supporting the theory with definitive experimental and clinical evidence. The persistent difference in operative morbidity and mortality and the better long-term survival after reparative procedures when compared with MVR, in chronic valve regurgitation,[20-26] encouraged David et al[14] to compare functional results between two groups of patients undergoing MVR with or without preservation of the subvalvular apparatus.

While LV end-diastolic, end-systolic, and stroke volumes decreased in both groups, there were significant differences in ejection fraction. Indeed, ejection fraction decreased only in patients undergoing traditional MVR, when evaluated at rest, while it increased significantly only in patients with preserved subvalvular apparatus, during exercise. Both LV systolic function (systolic pressure/end-systolic volume index) and LV performance (stroke volume index/end-diastolic volume index) were improved in patients with preserved subvalvular apparatus at rest and during exercise. The authors demonstrated how, in chronic mitral regurgitation, preop-erative LV ejection fraction can be misleadingly elevated due to the "low-impedance regurgitant jet."[3-6,27] On the other side this parameter is still relevant in clinical use because preoperative and postoperative variations are valuable in predicting operative and long-term outcomes.[14,28]

Based on his experience,[14,18] in 1986 David described the technique to preserve most chordal connections of both anterior and posterior leaflets during MVR.[29] The rationale was to produce a competent valve in which the natural chordal attachments were maintained in place, although partially relocated. Particular care was taken in selecting the prosthesis size since larger prostheses can increase the deleterious effect produced by the rigid prosthetic ring on the contractility of LV basal area.[30,31] Also David cautioned to avoid excess chordal tension. He recommended repositioning the stump of the anterior leaflet and oversewing the posterior one to prevent the rupture of papillary muscle heads or chordae tendineae and possible impingement on the prosthesis.[32-36]

In mitral stenosis, the positive influence of the subvalvular apparatus on LV function has been demonstrated comparing repair with traditional MVR.[37] The finding suggested that at least posterior chordae should be preserved

during MVR, with the additional reduction of the incidence of mid-ventricular wall rupture.[16,29,38] A substantial positive effect of chordal preservation in MVR was demonstrated by David and co-workers in ischemic mitral regurgitation as well.[39] While different parameters were significantly related with different end-points (preoperative cardiogenic shock with operative mortality, and ejection fraction < 35% with late mortality), complete excision of the valve and subvalvular apparatus was associated with both operative and late death with an actuarial survival of 89 ±9% versus 59 ±11% (preserved chordae tendineae versus completely excised valve) at 4-year follow-up. None of the other parameters related to the underlying ischemic pathology were significantly predictive of poor outcome. The authors concluded that it is critical to preserve the subvalvular apparatus, although altered by the ischemic injury. These data are consistent with those reported by Kay,[40,41] Waibel,[42] and Rankin[43,44] et al. Swanson and Starr[45] emphasized the importance of chordal preservation in MVR for ischemic regurgitation, while Cohn[46] confirmed the superiority of repair versus replacement, but could not find significant improvement in results when the subvalvular apparatus had been preserved or not in MVR. Moreover Goor et al[47] observed that the preservation of the posterior leaflet and chordae during MVR for ischemic valve incompetence is crucial to improve the results in a subgroup of particularly critical patients. Indeed when LV ejection fraction was ≤35%, operative and early mortality was 8/12 (67.7%) if the posterior leaflet had been resected, while it was 0/7 when it had been preserved. Moreover, low output syndrome was present in all 12 patients of the first group and in none of the second one.

Miki et al[15,48] confirmed the improvement with preservation of as much as possible of the papillary muscle-valve continuity: cardiac index, LV end-systolic volume index, LV ejection fraction and wall motion were significantly better when the subvalvular apparatus had been preserved. The various effects of complete valve preservation versus posterior leaflet and subvalvular apparatus preservation during MVR was accurately examined by Hennein and co-workers.[13] Three groups of patients were compared: (1) complete excision of the native valve, (2) complete mitral apparatus preservation, and (3) posterior leaflet apparatus preservation. Although the improvement in operative mortality was not statistically among the groups (probably due to the small number of events), all deaths occurred in the complete excision group (4/55). Survival analysis showed significantly better results for the preservation groups starting at the first year, and improvement in the NYHA functional class was statistically greater in the same patients. Functional parameters such as resting and exercise ejection fraction and treadmill exercise testing definitely improved with chordal preservation. Echocardiography demonstrated significant postoperative decrease in LV end-systolic dimension and maintenance of LV fractional shortening only when the valve apparatus had been preserved. The authors concluded that early and late results of MVR with preservation of the native valve apparatus were superior. However they asserted there was no significant difference between complete valve maintenance and preservation of the posterior leaflet apparatus alone, in case of mitral regurgitation.

Similar conclusions were reported by Tasdemir et al.[28] Patients randomly selected to undergo traditional MVR, or MVR with preservation of the posterior leaflet and chordae, demonstrated a significant difference in exercise ejection fraction between the two groups of patients, examined 18 months after operation. While ejection fraction significantly increased in response to effort in the preservation group, it decreased in patients undergoing traditional MVR, confirming the impairment of LV function produced by total removal of the mitral subvalvular apparatus. Also in this study the clinical relevance of ejection the fraction was validated, although preoperative values may be misleadingly elevated. Indeed low values correlated significantly with increased risk of irreversible postoperative congestive heart failure.[28] Preoperative ejection fraction, as an independent predictor of postoperative LV function, has been recently reported by Sarano.[26]

The effect of preserving the posterior valve apparatus during MVR was compared with the traditional MVR in two group of patients by Konstantinov et al.[49] Evaluating LV regional myocardial contraction, the authors observed significant improvement in the preservation group, interpreting this effect as secondary to increased myocardial compliance during the relaxation phase, rapid filling and pre-ejection.

Other authors recently analyzed different aspects of the influence of the subvalvular apparatus on LV function after MVR. Hofmeisteret al,[50] comparing patients undergoing mitral reconstruction with those undergoing MVR with preservation of papillary muscle-annulus continuity, showed that short and long axis fractional shortening was comparable. They concluded that preservation of the subvalvular apparatus during MVR preserves LV diastolic and systolic function as well as does mitral repair alone. Similar results were reported by Nagatsu et al[51] in a canine model. Preservation combined with MVR and satisfactory repair produces comparable effects on LV function, while inadequate repair is worse than valve replacement.

An interesting experimental study, performed by Ishihara et al,[52] evaluated the effect of MVR with chordal preservation on restoration of contractile function after the depression produced by chronic mitral regurgitation. In a canine model they produced severe mitral regurgitation and performed MVR with preservation of the subvalvular apparatus a few months later. Pulmonary capillary wedge pressure, forward stroke volume, end-systolic stress-volume relationship and end-systolic stiffness constant, significantly worsened by chronic regurgitation, returned to normal after chordal preservation and MVR, while ejection fraction increased with mitral regurgitation and decreased after MVR, but without statistical significance. Additionally the authors examined contraction characteristics of myocytes isolated at the end of the study; they observed normal extent and velocity of shortening. Recently also Spinale et al[53] reported the effects of long-standing mitral regurgitation, and subsequent MVR, on myocytes. They found an increase of myocyte size, associated with reduced myofibril content, after the experimental production of chronic regurgitation. Also the LV contractile state, expressed as end-systolic stiffness constant, was depressed. After MVR myofibril content and contractile state increased to normal values.

The efficacy of chordal preservation combined with MVR for mitral regurgitation in subgroups of patients with severely impaired left ventricular function was evaluated by Kaul, and Semenovski et al in two recent studies. Early and late mortality increased significantly in cases of depressed (< 25%) ejection fraction when the subvalvular apparatus had been completely excised (Group I), comparing with patients showing moderate depression of LV contractility (ejection fraction > 25%, mean 32%) and undergoing complete chordal excision (Group II), or severe depression, but with the subvalvular apparatus preserved (Group III). Similarly, actuarial survival and event-free curves, at 5 and 10 years, were significantly worse in Group I patients.[54] Ejection fraction increased and LV end-diastolic pressure decreased in patients with preserved subvalvular structures, while the opposite results were observed with chordal detachment.[55]

On the other hand Harpole et al[56] could not demonstrate a significant difference in postoperative LV function between patients undergoing traditional MVR and those in whom the subvalvular apparatus had been preserved. They based their research on the critical evaluation of previous reports, in which the conclusions had been drawn from the analysis of load-dependent variables. Therefore the authors also utilized load-independent parameters such as the stroke work/end-diastolic volume relationship, and LV end-systolic meridi-anal wall stress, obtained from two-dimensional Doppler echocardiograms. Significant differences were observed for LV ejection fraction and end-systolic meridianal wall stress, but only in cases of mitral regurgitation and never in mitral stenosis, while the differences in load-independent variables were not statistically significant. The authors de-emphasized the importance of preserving of the subvalvular apparatus to improve LV function during MVR. Yet as pointed in the editorial comment by Tyers,[57] this study, although accurate in the

analysis, is in some ways deficient. First, Harpole et al[56] defined as "standard MVR" the preservation of the posterior leaflets, while most surgeons still consider "traditional MVR" to include the excision of both leaflets and the subvalvular apparatus, as also performed by Harpole in almost half of his patients. Moreover only 12 patients were admitted to the study, and only 8 of them had mitral regurgitation, which benefits more from chordal preservation. In one of these eight patients the valve was completely excised, whereas in seven the posterior leaflet only was maintained. The significance of this study is reduced by these design flaws.

In a recent paper Okita et al[58] compared LV function in traditional MVR, chordal preserving MVR, and valve repair for mitral regurgitation. Early after operation, with cineangiography, they found significantly greater shortening of anterolateral and anterobasal areas, and of the long-axis in cases of chordal preserving versus traditional MVR. Valve repair produced a better result only in shortening of the diaphragmatic area. Reduction in global ejection fraction was comparable in all groups.

With mid-, long-term radionuclide angiography, the authors confirmed the differences in radial shortening of most LV areas with a concomitant better regional and global LV ejection fraction in patients with chordal preserving versus traditional MVR. Valve repair produced better results only in the inferolateral area. Also the region of papillary muscle insertion had significantly better contraction when chordal attachments had been preserved.

In a randomized study Horstkotte et al[59] compared two groups of patients undergoing isolated MVR with or without preservation of the posterior chordal apparatus. They found significantly better hemodynamic parameters and maximum exercise tolerance when chordae had been preserved. At follow-up there were fewer complications in this group of patients. These benefits were greater in cases of severe mitral regurgitation.

Many authors have suggested methods to improve subvalvular apparatus preservation during MVR.[15,29,38,60] Feikes et al[60] transpose anterior leaflet chordal attachments to the posterior annulus, trimming unsupported areas and debriding calcific nodules, to obtain uniform chordal tension and to avoid any possible interference with disk motion when a mechanical prosthesis is utilized. When a tilting disk prosthesis is utilized, it is oriented so the major orifice is facing the anterior annulus. Amano et al[38] described techniques in calcified stenotic mitral valve surgery. Before transposing posteriorly the two stumps of the anterior leaflet with their chordal attachments, the authors utilize an ultrasonic debridement tool to trim all the tissue to be transposed; then a tilting disk prosthesis is inserted, oriented in such a way as to carefully avoid any possible interference of the residual tissue with disk movements.

Although particular care is taken to prevent disk sticking, many cases of this often catastrophic event are reported, produced by residual tissue entrapment or papillary muscle rupture, due to excessive tension, and subsequent engagement with the tilting disk.[32-36] For this reason many authors suggested the use of only biological prostheses when part of the valve and a portion of the subvalvular apparatus are preserved.[14,19,29,39,46,54] Implantation of a biological prosthesis with preservation of the anterior mitral leaflet may produce left ventricular outflow tract obstruction due to the sail effect of redundant natural tissue.[61-64] In cases of severe impairment of cardiac function this complication requires reoperation to remove the obstructing leaflet.[62] In any case careful trimming of tissue from redundant myxomatous valves or debridement of fibrous and calcific nodules from rheumatic valves is required before insertion of any prosthesis.[13,15,29,32,46,54,56,60] Olinger[65] reported a case in which he was able to preserve the valve at reoperation, due to the degeneration of a bioprosthesis inserted six years earlier, and maintain the entire mitral apparatus. At reoperation the author repositioned the leaflets before inserting a new prosthesis.

These surgical maneuvers require surgical skill, take up precious aortic cross-clamp time and, in cases of massive alteration of valve structures, may be not be adequate to achieve a satisfactory and safe result. Therefore a few authors have suggested, in selected cases, complete removal of the native valve or preservation of mural chordae only, if not particularly altered, associated with the reconstruction of papillary muscle-annulus continuity with artificial chordae.[66-70] Bileaflet mechanical prostheses are then inserted in most of the cases. Although small series have only been reported so far, the preliminary clinical and echocardiographic data confirm the safety and efficacy of the technique. The deterioration of LV function, often observed after traditional MVR in patients with dysfunctional and dyskinetic ventricles for longstanding mitral stenosis, seems to be prevented by this artificial reconstruction of papillary muscle-annulus continuity.[68]

Vucinic[70] utilized this technique in 10 patients for heavy calcific stenotic mitral valve completely removed at the time of MVR. He performed cardiac catheterization in six of these patients 2 to 24 months after operation. Left ventricular global ejection fraction improved significantly. In particular, contractility was significantly increased in the anterolateral (base of the papillary muscle) and apical segments, confirming that restoration of papillary muscle-annular continuity is also beneficial in mitral stenosis or combined stenosis and insufficiency. In a few cases this artificial connection is reestablished only with the mural annulus, obtaining a satisfactory functional result and confirming the fundamental role of this part of the mitral apparatus in preserving the coordination of LV wall motion.[67,71-73]

PERSONAL EXPERIENCE

In the last 8 to 10 years rheumatic mitral pathology has almost disappeared in our country so most of our experience is based on degenerative mitral regurgitation, for which we perform mitral repair. In cases of mitral stenosis our policy has changed in the past few years. At the outset (1985-89) we performed many reparative procedures (besides commissurotomy), even in rheumatic stenosis. Calcium debridement, papillary and chordae splitting and chordae replacement with artificial chordae were often required expanding the indications to include the cases with severe involvement of the subvalvular apparatus.[74]

At follow-up we observed that these procedures did not prevent progression of pathological alterations leading to valve regurgitation. In fact we often observed progressive shrinkage of the leaflets with consequent central regurgitation due to loss of coaptation. For this reason since 1990 in cases of rheumatic disease, whenever complex procedures are required to obtain an acceptable result, we prefer to replace the valve. Our experience in mitral valve replacement is now based on these cases and on a few cases of degenerative disease in patients with associated complex pathologies requiring long aortic crossclamping time or elderly patients (>75 years). We attempt to avoid lengthy cardiopulmonary by-pass and patients with severe ischemic damage of the subvalvular apparatus. In all of these situations we completely preserve the connections of the posterior and commissural leaflets to the papillary muscles with any kind of prosthesis utilized. However, in a few situations, such as degenerative pathology with extensive rupture of posterior chordae or rheumatic cases with marked calcifications of the posterior leaflet and relative subvalvular apparatus, the preservation of these structures may cause difficulty in inserting the prosthesis. Therefore in these instances we prefer to remove the entire valve and subvalvular apparatus and to restore papillary-annulus continuity by the insertion of artificial chordae.

SURGICAL PROCEDURE

After removing both mitral leaflets and chordal connections to the papillary muscles, four 5-0 Gore-Tex® sutures are anchored to the papillary muscles in a "U" shape. Each side of the muscle is reinforced with one autologous pericardium pledget on (Fig. 10.1), as in case of artificial chordae insertion for mitral valve repair. The sutures are tied avoiding excessive tension with consequent papillary muscle head ischemia. The two strands of each suture are then fixed close each other in one of four points around the annulus—at the sites of two, four, eight and

ten o'clock—to distribute the stress uniformly (Fig. 10.2).

The length is set so that the artificial chordae are under tension with the relaxed heart. They are then tied and reinforced with autologous pericardium pledget. The prosthesis is inserted with interrupted "U" shaped sutures. The strands of the artificial chordae are passed through the annulus of the prosthesis as well (Fig. 10.3) to further reinforce it and are tied (Fig. 10.4). In a few cases (see clinical series) a small part of the posterior leaflet and associated chordae could be maintained and only two (four chordae) or three (six chordae) Gore-Tex® sutures were inserted.

CLINICAL SERIES

With the exception of one case performed in 1985, since 1990 we have inserted artificial chordae after complete removal of leaflets and subvalvular apparatus during mitral valve replacement in another 21 patients. Demographic and clinical data are reported in Table 10.1.

Table 1. Demographic and clinical data

Sex	
Male	13
Female	9
Age	
Mean	60.3
Range	44-75
Etiology	
Rheumatic	15
Degenerative	4
Ischemic	2
Infective	1
Mitral Lesion	
Stenosis	3
Insufficiency	7
Mixed	12
Associated Pathologies	
CAD	4
CAD + LV Aneurysm	1
AI + asc.ao. Aneurysm	1
AI + TI	1

CAD=coronary artery disease; LV=left ventricular; AI=aortic insufficiency; asc.ao.=ascending aorta; TI=tricuspid insufficiency.

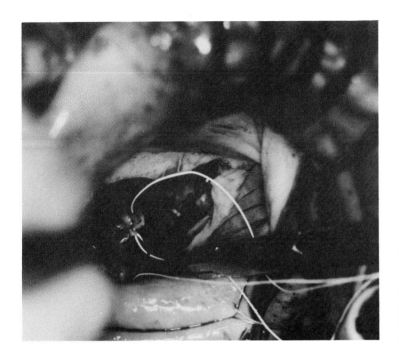

Fig. 10.1. After completely removing leaflets and chordae, four 5-0 Gore-Tex® stitches are anchored to the papillary muscles and are reinforced with treated autologous pericardium pledgets.

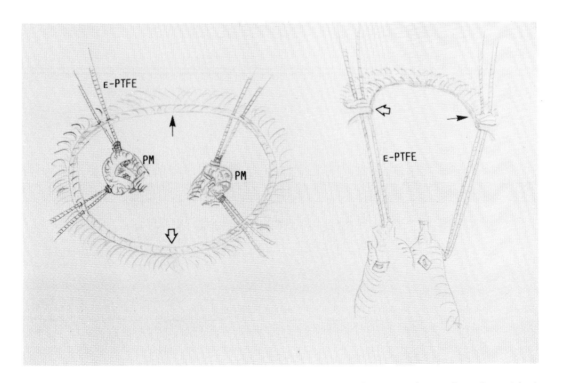

Fig. 10.2. The four pairs of artificial chordae are fixed to the mitral annulus at two, four, eight and ten o'clock. e-PTFE=artificial chordae; PM=papillary muscles; black arrow=anterior annulus; empty arrow=posterior annulus.

Table 2. Surgical procedure

Prosthesis
Biological	8
Mechanical	14

N. Artificial Chordae	N. Patients
4	4
6	2
8	16

Associated Procedures
CABG	4
CABG + LV Aneurysmectomy	1
AVR + asc.ao. Replacement	1
AVR + TVP	1

CABG=coronary artery by-pass grafting; LV=left ventricular; AVR=aortic valve replacement; asc.ao.=ascending aorta; TVP=tricuspid valve repair

The mean age was higher than that of the patients undergoing mitral repair. In the great majority of the cases the etiology was rheumatic and the lesion produced was combined mitral stenosis and insufficiency.

A bileaflet mechanical prosthesis was inserted in 14 cases, while in 8 cases a bioprosthesis was utilized. In 16 patients eight artificial chordae (four Gore-Tex® sutures) were inserted, in two patients six chordae and in four patients four chordae. The associated procedures are described in Table 10.2.

All patients survived the operation and were discharged from the hospital. No chordae-related complications were reported during a mean follow-up of 18.2 months (range 3-96 months).

The patient operated in 1985 has been recently reoperated due to degeneration of the bioprosthesis inserted at the first operation. Artificial chordae, still in place, were completely covered by a fibrous sheath and were under tension with the heart relaxed. They were left in place at reoperation when

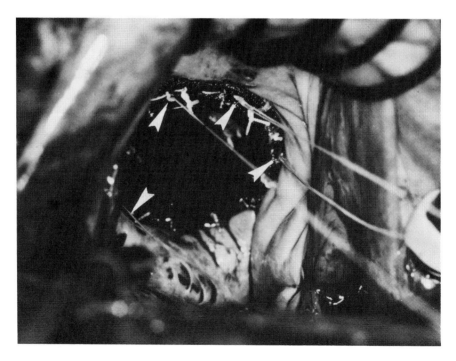

Fig. 10.3. After inserting the artificial prosthesis the two strands of each suture utilized as artificial chorda are passed through the prosthesis sewing ring and tied (arrows).

a new bioprosthesis was inserted (the patient is 75 years old), and consequently no histologic examination could be performed.

No other valve-related complications have been reported so far. Echocardiography performed at 6 and 12 months and then once a year confirmed that the artificial chordae were acting to reduce ventricular deformation after mitral valve replacement. No impingement on the prostheses could be demonstrated since they retained tension throughout the cardiac cycle and they are placed far from the area of movement of the mechanical disk.

This technique, although utilized in a small number of patients, is safe and reliable. It permits restoration of the papillary muscle-annular continuity once it is interrupted as with the inevitable removal of all chordae. Indeed with eight chordae inserted around the circumference of the orifice the stress is uniformly distributed. Also this procedure saves time when compared with other techniques that require calcium debridement and partial leaflet repositioning in cases of calcified stenotic mitral valve.

REFERENCES

1. Lillehei CW. Discussion of: Hennein HA, Swain JA, McIntosh CL et al: Comparative assessment of chordal preservation versus chordal resection during mitral valve replacement. J Thorac Cardiovasc Surg 1990; 99:828-37.

2. Lillehei CW, Levy MJ, Bonnabeau RC. Mitral valve replacement with preservation of the papillary muscles and the chordae tendineae. J Thorac Cardiovasc Surg 1964; 47:532-43.

3. Rankin JS, Nicholas LM, Kouchoukos NT. Experimental mitral regurgitation: Effects on left ventricular function before and after elimination of chronic regurgitation in the dog. J Thorac Cardiovasc Surg 1975; 70:478-88.

4. Wong CYH, Spotnitz HM. Systolic and diastolic properties of the human left ventricle during valve replacement for chronic mitral regurgitation. Am J Cardiol 1981; 47:40-50.

5. Urschel CW, Covell JW, Sonnenblick EH et al. Myocardial mechanics in aortic and

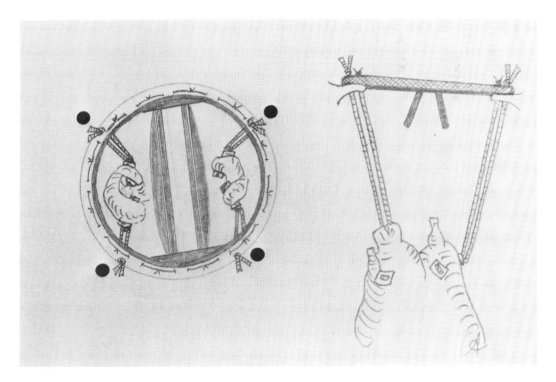

Fig. 10.4. Schematic illustration of the final appearance in cases of mitral valve replacement with a bileaflet mechanical prosthesis and four pairs of artificial chordae (black dots).

mitral valvular regurgitation. The concept of instantaneous impedance as a determinant of the performance of the intact heart. J Clin Invest 1968; 47:867-83.

6. Rozich J, Carabello B, Usher B et al. A mechanism by which ejection performance is preserved following mitral valve repair but not replacement for chronic mitral regurgitation. Circulation 1991; 84 (Suppl II):II 578.

7. Kennedy JW, Doces JG, Stewart DK. Left ventricular function before and following surgical treatment of mitral valve disease. Am Heart J 1979; 97:592-8.

8. Boucher CA, Bingham JB, Osbakken MD et al. Early changes in left ventricular size and function after correction of ventricular volume overload. Am J Cardiol 1981; 47:991-1004.

9. Huikuri HV. Effect of mitral valve replacement on left ventricular function in mitral regurgitation. Br Heart J 1983; 49:328-33.

10. Carabello BA. The mitral valve apparatus: Is there still room to doubt the importance of its preservation? J Heart Valve Dis 1993; 2:250-2.

11. Bjork VO, Bjork L, Malers E. Left ventricular function after resection of the papillary muscles in patients with total mitral valve replacement. J Thorac Cardiovasc Surg 1964; 48:635-9.

12. Rastelli GC, Tsakiris AG, Frye RL et al. Exercise tolerance and haemodynamic studies after replacement of canine mitral valve with and without preservation of chordae tendineae. Circulation 1967; 35 (Suppl I):I 34-I 39.

13. Hennein HA, Swain JA, McIntosh CL et al. Comparative assessment of chordal preservation versus chordal resection during mitral valve replacement. J Thorac Cardiovasc Surg 1990; 99:828-37.

14. David TE, Burns RJ, Bacchus CM et al. Mitral valve replacement for mitral regurgitation with and without preservation of chordae tendineae. J Thorac Cardiovasc Surg 1984; 88:718-25.

15. Miki S, Kusuhara K, Ueda Y et al. Mitral valve replacement with preservation of chordae tendineae and papillary muscles. Ann Thorac Surg 1988; 45:28-34.

16. Miller Jr DW, Johnson DD, Ivey TD. Does preservation of the posterior chordae tendineae enhance survival during mitral valve replacement? Ann Thorac Surg 1979; 28:22-7.

17. David TE, Strauss AD, Mesher E et al. Is it important to preserve the chordae tendineae and papillary muscles during mitral valve replacement? Can J Surg 1981; 24:236-9.

18. David TE, Uden DE, Strauss HD. The importance of the mitral apparatus in left ventricular function after correction of mitral regurgitation. Circulation 1983; 68 (Suppl II):II 76-II 82.

19. Hetzer R, Bougiokas G, Franz M et al. Mitral valve replacement with preservation of papillary muscles and chordae tendineae: Revival of a seemingly forgotten concept. I. Preliminary clinical report. Thorac Cardiovasc Surg 1983; 31:291-6.

20. Marshall Jr WG, Kouchoukos NT, Karp RB et al. Late results after mitral valve replacement with the Bjork-Shiley and porcine prostheses. J Thorac Cardiovasc Surg 1983; 85:902-10.

22. Chaffin JS, Daggett WM. Mitral valve replacement. A nine-year follow-up of risks and survival. Ann Thorac Surg 1979; 27:312-9.

23. Yacoub M, Halim M, Radley-Smith R et al. Surgical treatment of mitral regurgitation caused by floppy valves. Repair versus replacement. Circulation 1981; 64 (Suppl II):II 210-II 216.

24. Carpentier A, Chauvaud S, Fabiani JN et al. Reconstructive surgery of mitral incompetence. Ten-year appraisal. J Thorac Cardiovasc Surg 1980; 79:338-48.

25. Shore DF, Wong P, Paneth M. Valve repair versus replacement in the surgical management of ruptured chordae. A postoperative echocardiographic assessment of mitral valve function. J Cardiovasc Surg 1982; 23:378-82.

26. Sarano ME, McGoon MD, Orszulak TA et al. Clinical and echocardiographic predictors of left ventricular function after mitral regurgitation surgery. Circulation 1992; 86 (Suppl I):I 724.

27. Braunwald E. Mitral regurgitation physiological, clinical, surgical considerations. N

Engl J Med 1969; 281:425-33.

28. Tasdemir O, Katircioglu F, Catav Z et al. Clinical results of mitral valve replacement with and without preservation of the posterior mitral valve leaflet and subvalvular apparatus. J Cardiovasc Surg 1991; 32:509-15.

29. David TE. Mitral valve replacement with preservation of chordae tendineae: Rationale and technical considerations. Ann Thorac Surg 1986; 41:680-2.

30. Spence PA, Peniston CM, David TE et al. Toward a better understanding of the etiology of left ventricular dysfunction after mitral valve replacement: An experimental study with possible clinical implications. Ann Thorac Surg 1986; 41:363-71.

31. Sakai K, Sakaki S, Hirata N et al. Assessment of postoperative left ventricular function after mitral valve repair for mitral regurgitation. Circulation 1991; 84 (Suppl II):II 578.

32. Trites PN, Kiser JC, Johnson C et al. Occlusion of Medtronic-Hall mitral valve prosthesis by ruptured papillary muscle and chordae tendineae. J Thorac Cardiovasc Surg 1984; 88:301-2.

33. Masters RG, Keon WJ. Extrinsic obstruction of the Medtronic-Hall disk valve in the mitral position. Ann Thorac Surg 1988; 45:210-2.

34. Pai GP, Ellison RG, Rubin JW et al. Disk immobilization of Bjork-Shiley and Medtronic Hall valves during and immediately after valve replacement. Ann Thorac Surg 1987; 44:73-6.

35. Hall KV. Surgical considerations for avoiding disc interference based on ten year experience with the Medtronic Hall heart valve. J Cardiac Surg 1988; 3:103-8.

36. Mok CK, Cheung DLC, Chiu CSW et al. An unusual lethal complication of preservation of chordae tendineae in mitral valve replacement. J Thorac Cardiovasc Surg 1988; 95:534-6.

37. Kazama S, Nishiguchi K, Sonoda K et al. Postoperative left ventricular function in patients with mitral stenosis. The effect of commissurotomy and valve replacement on left ventricular systolic function. Jpn Heart J 1986; 27:35-42.

38. Amano J, Fujiwara H, Sugano T et al. Modified preservation of all annular-papillary continuity in replacement of the calcified mitral valve. Thorac Cardiovasc Surgeon 1992; 40:79-81.

39. David TE, Ho WC. The effect of preservation of chordae tendineae on mitral valve replacement for postinfarction mitral regurgitation. Circulation 1986; 74 (Suppl I):I 116-I 120.

40. Kay JH, Zubiate P, Mendez MA et al. Surgical treatment of mitral insufficiency secondary to coronary artery disease. J Thorac Cardiovasc Surg 1980; 79:12-8.

41. Kay GL, Kay JH, Zubiate P et al. Mitral valve repair for mitral regurgitation secondary to coronary artery disease. Circulation 1987; 78 (Suppl I):I 88-I 98.

42. Waibel AW, Hausdorf G, Vetter HO et al. Results of surgical therapy in ischemic mitral regurgitation. In: Vetter HO, Hetzer R, Schmutzler H, eds. Ischemic mitral incompetence. Darmstadt: Steinkopff Verlag, New York: Springer Verlag, 1991:149-56.

43. Rankin JS, Hickey MSJ, Smith LR et al. Current concepts in the pathogenesis and treatment of ischemic mitral regurgitation. In: Vetter HO, Hetzer R, Schmutzler H, eds. Ischemic mitral incompetence. Darmstadt: Steinkopff Verlag, New York: Springer Verlag, 1991:157-78.

44. Rankin JS, Livesey SA, Smith LR et al. Trends in the surgical treatment of ischemic mitral regurgitation: Effects of mitral valve repair on hospital mortality. Semin Thorac Cardiovasc Surg 1989; 1:149-63.

45. Swanson JS, Starr A. Surgical results with severe ischemic mitral regurgitation. In: Vetter HO, Hetzer R, Schmutzler H, eds. Ischemic mitral incompetence. Darmstadt: Steinkopff Verlag, New York: Springer Verlag, 1991: 187-93.

46. Cohn LH. Surgical treatment of ischemic mitral regurgitation by repair and replacement. In: Vetter HO, Hetzer R, Schmutzler H, eds. Ischemic mitral incompetence. Darmstadt: Steinkopff Verlag, New York: Springer Verlag, 1991: 179-86.

47. Goor DA, Mohr R, Lavee J et al. Preservation of the posterior leaflet during mechanical valve replacement for ischemic mitral regurgitation and complete myocardial

revascularization. J Thorac Cardiovasc Surg 1988; 96:253-60.

48. Miki S, Kusuhara K, Ueda Y et al. Mitral valve replacement with preservation of whole papillary muscles and chordae tendineae. J Cardiovasc Surg (Torino) 1985; 26 (Suppl):3.

49. Konstantinov BA, Iakolev VF, Tarichko IV et al. Effect of preserved subvalvular apparatus on regional left ventricular function after mitral valve prosthesis in patients operated on for mitral insufficiency. Vestn Akad Med Nauk SSSR 1990; 10:3-6.

50. Hofmeister J, Siniawski H, Warnekke H et al. Mitral valve replacement and preservation of the mitral apparatus. Proceedings Medtronic Cardiovascular Technology Symposium, Ayrshire, Scotland, October 24-27, 1991.

51. Nagatsu M, Ishihara K, DeFreyte G et al. Mitral valve repair versus chordae-sparing mitral valve replacement in dogs with contractile dysfunction due to experimental mitral regurgitation. Circulation 1992; 86 (Suppl I):I 699.

52. Ishihara K, Zile MR, Kanazawa S et al. Left ventricular mechanics and myocyte function after correction of experimental chronic mitral regurgitation by combined mitral valve replacement and preservation of the native mitral valve apparatus. Circulation 1992; 86 (Suppl II):II 16-II 25.

53. Spinale F, Ishihara K, Zile M et al. The structural basis for changes in LV function due to chronic mitral regurgitation following correction of the volume overload. Circulation 1992; 86 (Suppl I):I 698.

54. Kaul TK, Ramsdale DR, Meek D et al. Mitral valve replacement in patients with severe mitral regurgitation and impaired left ventricular function. Int J Cardiol 1992; 35:169-79.

55. Semenovski ML, Sokolov VV, Chestukhin. Hemodynamic evaluation of the effectiveness of preservation of subvalvular structures in mitral valve prosthesis. Grud Serdechnososudistaia Khir 1990; 9:21-6.

56. Harpole Jr DH, Rankin S, Wolfe WG et al. Effects of standard mitral valve replacement on left ventricular function. Ann Thorac Surg 1990; 49:866-74.

57. Tyers GFO. Mitral valve replacement: What should be the standard technique. Ann

Thorac Surg 1990; 49:861-2.

58. Okita Y, Miki S, Kusuhara K et al. Analysis of left ventricular motion after mitral valve replacement with a technique of preservation of all chordae tendineae. Comparison with conventional mitral valve replacement or mitral valve repair. J Thorac Cardiovasc Surg 1992; 104:786-95.

59. Horstkotte D, Schulte HD, Bircks W et al. The effect of chordal preservation on late outcome after mitral valve replacement: A randomized study. J Heart Valve Dis 1993; 2:150-8.

60. Feikes HL, Daugharthy JB, Perry JE et al. Preservetion of all chordae tendineae and papillary muscle during mitral valve replacement with a tilting disc valve. J Cardiac Surg 1990; 5:81-5.

61. Come PC, Riley MF, Weintraub RM et al. Dynamic left ventricular outflow tract obstruction when the anterior leaflet is retained at prosthetic mitral valve replacement. Ann Thorac Surg 1987; 43:561-3.

62. Reed MK, Iverson LIG. Simplified correction of outflow obstruction after mitral valve replacement. Ann Thorac Surg 1992; 54:985-6.

63. Jacobs LE, Kotler MN, Ioli A. Left ventricular outflow tract obstruction following mitral valve replacement with Carpentier-Edwards prosthesis. Echocardiography 1990; 7:147-53.

64. Roberts WC, Dollar AL. Extreme obstruction to left ventricular outflow by a bioprosthesis in the mitral valve position. Am Heart J 1991; 121:607-8.

65. Olinger GN. Rereplacement of the mitral valve with preservation of the subvalvular apparatus. Ann Thorac Surg 1992; 54:188-90.

66. David TE. Mitral valve replacement with preservation of chordae tendineae. Saudi Heart J 1990; 1:32-6.

67. Bernhard A, Sievers HH, Nellesen U et al. Improved mitral valve replacement. Eur J Cardio-Thorac Surg 1990; 4:224-5.

68. Okita Y, Miki S, Ueda Y et al. Artificial chordal reconstruction using expanded polytetrafluoroethylene (ePTFE) sutures for mitral valve replacement in patients with mitral stenosis. Proceedings 6th Annual

Meeting of the European Association for Cardio-Thoracic Surgery, Geneva, Switzerland, September 14-16, 1992:pg 114.

69. Bonchek LI. "Chordal" preservation during mitral valve rereplacement. Ann Thorac Surg 1993; 55:196-200.

70. Vucinic M. Suspension of the papillary muscles during valve replacement for mitral stenosis. J Heart Valve Dis 1993; 2:311-3.

71. Rushmer RF, Finlayson BL, Nash AA. Movements of the mitral valve. Circ Res 1956; 4:337-42.

72. Hagl S, Heimisch H, Meisner H et al. In-situ function of the papillary muscles in the intact canine left ventricle. In: Duran C, Angell WW, Johnson AD, Oury JH, eds. Recent progress in mitral valve disease. London: Butterworths, 1984:397-409.

73. Hansen DE, Cahill PD, Derby GC et al. Relative contributions of the anterior and posterior mitral chordae tendineae to canine global left ventricular systolic performance. J Thorac Cardiovasc Surg 1987; 93:45-55.

74. Zussa C, Frater RWM, Polesel E et al. Artificial mitral valve chordae: Experimental and clinical experience. Ann Thorac Surg 1990; 50:367-73.

=CHAPTER 11=

CONCLUSIONS

Our experience with e-PTFE sutures utilized as chordae substitutes in mitral valve repair or replacement is in the seventh year. More than 100 cases of valve repair and more than 20 of valve replacement have been successfully treated with artificial chordae insertion so far. After a short learning period in which a small number of artificial chordae were inserted with less than optimal results in a few instances, our increasing confidence in this technique resulted in a greater number of chordae inserted and in a consequent improvement of the results.

Also we had many opportunities to discuss our results with Dr. Tirone David who has had a similar successful experience in Toronto.

In fact operative risk is very low, independent of the etiology, clinical conditions and age of the patient. The rate of artificial chordae-related complications is negligible. So far there has been one transitory ischemic attack and one reoperation due to an error in tying e-PTFE sutures. No signs of material degradation or calcification could be detected and morphologic characteristics of the sutures were stable throughout follow-up.

A few final considerations should be emphasized. First, the long-term result of any reparative procedure on the mitral valve is strictly correlated with the etiology of valve disease. It is our opinion that rheumatic cases should be repaired only if leaflet tissue is still pliable and without signs of active disease, mostly in aged patients. For this reason accurate preoperative echocardiography of the mitral apparatus is essential to predict the feasibility of repair and to establish the timing of operation, since in cases of probable valve replacement the operation should be deferred until the patient is in NYHA functional class III. On the other hand, in cases of degenerative pathology the great likelihood of valve repair should suggest early referral for surgery, before any left ventricular impairment, independent of the functional class.

Second, artificial chordae represent one more tool for cardiac surgeons. It is not intended to replace other satisfactory traditional techniques, but it should supplement those that cannot otherwise yield completely adequate results. In particular, when diffuse chordal pathology suggests possible progression of valve disease, artificial chordae should be utilized to prevent this progresion and to"stabilize" the subvalvular apparatus anatomy.

Third, current techniques of myocardial protection extend the safe period of ischemia. This permits expansion of the indications to include cases of diffuse change of the chordal apparatus requiring various surgical maneuvers and several artificial chordae to achieve an optimal result. For instance, in our experience, fibroelastic deficiency with a great number of very thin, elongated chordae arising from several slim papillary muscles in the presence of attenuated leaflet tissue are very difficult to correct with traditional techniques. In these cases we prefer to insert many artificial chordae to restore the correct position of the leaflets. The time "wasted" inserting several pairs of artificial chordae is worthwhile since the outcome is better and durable.

In elderly patients we think that this procedure, although time consuming, is very advantageous since the benefits of valve preservation accruing to ventricular performance overcome concern about the extension of ischemic time. Moreover within a certain range, increased ischemia time has been shown not to increase operative risk in these patients, provided excellent myocardial protection is achieved.

In conclusion, we recommend utilization of e-PTFE chordae in cases of:

1. diffuse fibroelastic deficiency;
2. rupture of anterior chordae associated with posterior prolapse or flail leaflet;
3. flail posterior leaflet too extensive to be corrected with a large quadrangular resection;
4. diffuse myxomatous degeneration, with supportive function to prevent further progression of the pathology;
5. isolated thick or calcified chordae that reduce leaflet mobility, although in the presence of flexible cusp tissue;
6. commissural tissue prolapse produced by extensive commissurotomy;
7. valve replacement when it is impossible to preserve at least the posterior subvalvular apparatus.

In these situations the results are quite satisfactory and after a short learning period the technique becomes absolutely reliable and reproducible. It permits the repair of more mitral valves and improves ventricular function in cases of mitral valve replacement when removal of the subvalvular apparatus is necessary.

INDEX